Evidence Synthesis
Number 108

Vitamin, Mineral, and Multivitamin Supplements for the Primary Prevention of Cardiovascular Disease and Cancer: A Systematic Evidence Review for the U.S. Preventive Services Task Force

Prepared for:
Agency for Healthcare Research and Quality
U.S. Department of Health and Human Services
540 Gaither Road
Rockville, MD 20850
www.ahrq.gov

Contract No. HHSA 290-2007-10057-I

Prepared by:
Kaiser Permanente Research Affiliates Evidence-based Practice Center
Kaiser Permanente Center for Health Research
Portland, OR

Investigators:
Stephen P. Fortmann, MD
Brittany U. Burda, MPH
Caitlyn A. Senger, MPH
Jennifer S. Lin, MD, MCR
Tracy L. Beil, MS
Elizabeth O'Connor, PhD
Evelyn P. Whitlock, MD, MPH

AHRQ Publication No. 14-05199-EF-1
November 2013

Note: A journal article associated with this work was published in *Annals of Internal Medicine*. At the request of the journal, we featured fixed effects models for pooled outcomes reported in the manuscript. The fixed effects models produced very small changes compared with the random effects models and do not change the overall findings of the report. **Appendix H** provides a comparison between the fixed effects and random effects model results for selected outcomes.

This report is based on research conducted by the Kaiser Permanente Research Affiliates Evidence-based Practice Center (EPC) under contract to the Agency for Healthcare Research and Quality (AHRQ), Rockville, MD (Contract No. HHSA 290-2007-10057-I). The findings and conclusions in this document are those of the authors, who are responsible for its contents; the findings and conclusions do not necessarily represent the views of AHRQ. Therefore, no statement in this report should be construed as an official position of AHRQ or of the U.S. Department of Health and Human Services.

The information in this report is intended to help health care decisionmakers—patients and clinicians, health system leaders, and policymakers, among others—make well-informed decisions and thereby improve the quality of health care services. This report is not intended to be a substitute for the application of clinical judgment. Anyone who makes decisions concerning the provision of clinical care should consider this report in the same way as any medical reference and in conjunction with all other pertinent information; that is, in the context of available resources and circumstances presented by individual patients.

This report may be used, in whole or in part, as the basis for development of clinical practice guidelines and other quality enhancement tools, or as a basis for reimbursement and coverage policies. AHRQ or U.S. Department of Health and Human Services endorsement of such derivative products may not be stated or implied.

This document is in the public domain and may be used and reprinted without permission except those copyrighted materials that are clearly noted in the document. Further reproduction of those copyrighted materials is prohibited without the specific permission of copyright holders.

Acknowledgments

The authors gratefully acknowledge the following individuals for their contributions to this project: Robert McNellis, MPH, PA-C, at AHRQ; Virginia Moyer, MD, MPH, Michael LeFevre, MD, MSPH, and Wanda Nicholson, MD, MPH, MBA, of the U.S. Preventive Services Task Force; JoAnn Manson, MD, DrPH, MPH, Thomas Trikalinos, MD, PhD, and Janelle Peralez-Gunn, MPH, for providing expert review; and Carin M. Olson, MD, MS, Daphne Plaut, MLS, and Heather Baird at the Kaiser Permanente Center for Health Research.

Suggested Citation

Fortmann SP, Burda BU, Senger CA, Lin J, Beil T, O'Connor E, Whitlock EP. Vitamin, Mineral, and Multivitamin Supplements for the Primary Prevention of Cardiovascular Disease and Cancer: A Systematic Evidence Review for the U.S. Preventive Services Task Force.

Evidence Report No. 108. AHRQ Publication No. 14-05199-EF-1. Rockville, MD: Agency for Healthcare Research and Quality; 2013.

Structured Abstract

Background: In the United States, dietary supplements are commonly used to prevent chronic diseases, including cardiovascular disease (CVD) and cancer.

Purpose: To systematically review evidence for the use of multivitamins or single nutrients and functionally related nutrient pairs for the prevention of CVD and cancer in the general population (primary prevention).

Methods: We searched MEDLINE, EMBASE, Cochrane Database of Systematic Reviews, the Database of Abstracts of Reviews of Effects, and Cochrane Central Register of Controlled Trials to identify literature that was published between 2005 and January 29, 2013. We also examined the references from the previous reviews and other relevant reviews to identify additional studies; we also searched Web sites of government agencies and other organizations for grey literature. Two investigators independently reviewed identified abstracts and full-text articles against a set of a priori inclusion and quality criteria. One investigator abstracted data into an evidence table and a second investigator checked these data. We qualitatively and quantitatively synthesized the results for the four key questions and grouped the included studies by study supplement. We conducted meta-analyses using Mantel-Haenzel fixed effects models for overall cancer incidence, CVD incidence, and all-cause mortality.

Results: We included 103 articles representing 26 unique studies. Very few studies examined the use of multivitamin supplements. Two trials showed a protective effect against cancer in men; only one of these trials included women and found no effect. No effects of treatment were seen on CVD or all-cause mortality. Beta-carotene showed a negative effect on lung cancer incidence and mortality among individuals at high risk for lung cancer at baseline (i.e., smokers and asbestos-exposed workers); this effect was persistent even when combined with vitamin A or E. Trials of vitamin E supplementation showed mixed results and altogether had no overall effect on cancer, CVD, or all-cause mortality. Only one of two included selenium trials showed a beneficial effect for colorectal and prostate cancer; however, this trial included a small sample size. The few studies addressing folic acid, vitamin C, and vitamin A showed no effect on CVD, cancer, and mortality. Vitamin D and/or calcium supplementation also showed no overall effect on CVD, cancer, and mortality. Harms were infrequently reported and aside from limited paradoxical effects for some supplements, were not considered serious.

Conclusions: There are a limited number of trials examining the effects of dietary supplements on the primary prevention of CVD and cancer; the majority showed no effect in healthy populations. Clinical heterogeneity of included studies limits generalizability of results to the general primary care population. Results from trials in at-risk populations discourage additional studies for particular supplements (e.g., beta-carotene); however, future research in general primary care populations and on other supplements is required to address research gaps.

Table of Contents

Chapter 1. Introduction 1
  Scope and Purpose 1
  Background 1
    Vitamins and Minerals 1
    Regulation of Dietary Supplements in the United States 1
    Use of Vitamin and Mineral Supplements in the United States 2
    Current Clinical Practice in the United States 2
    Prevalence and Burden of CVD and Cancer in the United States 3
    Traditional Risk Factors and Common Pathologic Mechanisms for CVD and Cancer 4
    Role of Vitamins and Minerals in the Prevention of CVD and Cancer 4
  Previous USPSTF Recommendation 6
Chapter 2. Methods 7
  Key Questions and Analytic Framework 7
  Data Sources and Searches 7
  Study Selection 8
  Quality Assessment 9
  Data Extraction 10
  Data Synthesis and Analysis 11
  USPSTF Involvement 12
Chapter 3. Results 13
  Literature Search 13
  KQ 1. What Is the Efficacy of Multivitamin Supplement Use on Health Outcomes in the General Adult Population? 13
  KQ 2. What Is Known About the Safety of Multivitamin Supplement Use in the General Adult Population? 13
    Summary of Results 13
    Study Details 14
    CVD 15
    Cancer 15
    All-Cause Mortality 16
    Harms 16
  KQ 3. What Is the Efficacy of Supplementation With Single Nutrients or Functionally Related Nutrient Pairs on Health Outcomes in the General Adult Population? 17
  KQ 4. What Is Known About the Safety of Single Nutrient Use in the General Adult Population? 17
    Beta-Carotene 18
    Vitamin E 21
    Selenium 24
    Vitamin A 26
    Vitamin C 28
    Folic Acid 29
    Vitamin D 30
    Vitamin D and Calcium 32

    Calcium 33
    Summary of Pooled Data 35
Chapter 4. Discussion 37
    Summary of Evidence 37
    Limitations in the Body of Evidence 40
    Limitations in Our Approach 42
    Applicability 43
    Future Research 44
    Conclusions 45
References 47

Figures
Figure 1. Analytic Framework
Figure 2. Relative Risk for Any Cardiovascular Disease Incidence at Longest Followup Only, by Supplement
Figure 3. Relative Risk for Any Cancer Incidence at Longest Followup Only, by Supplement
Figure 4. Relative Risk for All-Cause Mortality at Longest Followup Only, by Supplement

Tables
Table 1. Dietary Reference Intake Definitions
Table 2. Vitamin and Mineral Supplement Use in the United States, NHANES 2003–2006
Table 3. Recommendations of Other Organizations
Table 4. Framingham Heart Study Average Annual Incidence Rates of Cardiovascular Disease in the United States, 1980–2003
Table 5. Centers for Disease Control and Prevention Age-Adjusted Mortality Rates of Cardiovascular Disease in the United States Based on I00-I99 Codes, 2009
Table 6. SEER Incidence Rates of Cancer in the United States, 2005–2009
Table 7. SEER Mortality Rates of Cancer in the United States, 2005–2009
Table 8. Multivitamin Evidence Summary
Table 9. Vitamin and Mineral Components of the Multivitamin Studies
Table 10. Cardiovascular Disease Incidence and Mortality Among Multivitamin Studies
Table 11. Cancer Incidence and Mortality Among Multivitamin Studies
Table 12. All-Cause Mortality Among Multivitamin Studies
Table 13. Beta-Carotene Evidence Summary
Table 14. Cardiovascular Disease Incidence and Mortality Among Beta-Carotene Studies
Table 15. Cancer Incidence and Mortality Among Beta-Carotene Studies
Table 16. All-Cause Mortality Among Beta-Carotene Studies
Table 17. Yellowing of the Skin Among Beta-Carotene Studies
Table 18. Vitamin E Evidence Summary
Table 19. Cardiovascular Disease Incidence and Mortality Among Vitamin E Studies
Table 20. Cancer Incidence and Mortality Among Vitamin E Studies
Table 21. All-Cause Mortality Among Vitamin E Studies
Table 22. Selenium Evidence Summary
Table 23. Cardiovascular Disease Incidence and Mortality Among Selenium Studies
Table 24. Cancer Incidence and Mortality Among Selenium Studies
Table 25. All-Cause Mortality Among Selenium Studies

Table 26. Vitamin A Evidence Summary
Table 27. Vitamin C Evidence Summary
Table 28. Cardiovascular Disease Incidence and Mortality Among Vitamin C Studies
Table 29. Cancer Incidence and Mortality Among Vitamin C Studies
Table 30. All-Cause Mortality Among Vitamin C Studies
Table 31. Folic Acid Evidence Summary
Table 32. Vitamin D Evidence Summary
Table 33. Cardiovascular Disease Incidence and Mortality Among Vitamin D Studies
Table 34. Cancer Incidence and Mortality Among Vitamin D Studies
Table 35. All-Cause Mortality Among Vitamin D Studies
Table 36. Vitamin D and Calcium Evidence Summary
Table 37. Cardiovascular Disease Incidence and Mortality Among Combined Vitamin D and Calcium Supplement Studies
Table 38. Cancer Incidence and Mortality Among Combined Vitamin D and Calcium Supplement Studies
Table 39. All-Cause Mortality Among Combined Vitamin D and Calcium Supplement Studies
Table 40. Calcium Evidence Summary
Table 41. Cardiovascular Disease Incidence and Mortality Among Calcium Studies
Table 42. Cancer Incidence and Mortality Among Calcium Studies
Table 43. All-Cause Mortality Among Calcium Alone vs. Placebo Studies
Table 44. Summary of Evidence of Included Studies

Appendixes
Appendix A. Dietary Reference Intakes
Appendix B. Detailed Methods
Appendix C. Ongoing Studies
Appendix D. Excluded Studies
Appendix E. Evidence Tables
Appendix F. Outcomes Reported by Original Randomized Arms Among the 2x2 Factorial-Designed Randomized, Controlled Trials
Appendix G. Additional Meta-Analysis Figures
Appendix H. Sensitivity Analysis: Random vs. Fixed Effects Models

Chapter 1. Introduction

Scope and Purpose

We conducted this systematic review to help the Agency for Healthcare Research and Quality (AHRQ) update its recommendation on the use of multivitamins for the prevention of cardiovascular disease (CVD) and cancer in the general population. The U.S. Preventive Services Task Force (USPSTF) will use this review to update its 2003 recommendations on routine vitamin supplementation to prevent chronic diseases.[1] This review addresses the benefits and harms of single, paired, and multiple vitamins and/or minerals as primary prevention for CVD and cancer in the general population without nutritional deficiencies or existing chronic diseases.

Background

Vitamins and Minerals

Vitamins (e.g., vitamin A, B, C, D, and E) are organic compounds that are essential to maintaining health. Minerals, on the other hand, are inorganic substances that humans need to maintain their health (e.g., calcium, iron, zinc).[2] Multivitamin and/or multimineral supplements contain three or more vitamins and/or minerals without herbs, hormones, or drugs. The U.S. Food and Nutrition Board of the Institute of Medicine has also determined that each of these components is present at a dose less than the tolerable upper intake level.[2-8] We refer to multivitamin/multimineral supplements as multivitamins because this is how they are marketed and sold. We do not consider other essential nutrients, such as essential fatty acids, to be vitamins or minerals.

Between 1941 and 1994, the Recommended Dietary Allowances (RDAs) of the United States and the Dietary Standards/Recommended Nutrient Intakes (RNIs) of Canada dictated the nutrition polices of their respective countries. By the 1990s, however, concerns about the accuracy of the RDAs and RNIs in both countries arose as nutritional research advanced and measurement of nutrients improved. In 1997, the Food and Nutrition Board published a broader set of dietary reference values called Dietary Reference Intakes (DRIs). DRIs expanded upon and replaced RDAs and RNIs with four categories of intakes intended to help individuals optimize their health, prevent disease, and avoid consuming too much of a specific nutrient (**Table 1**).[2]

Most commercially available supplements generally contain vitamins and/or minerals at doses that are close to the recommended dietary allowance, but are still below the tolerable upper intake levels set by the U.S. Food and Nutrition Board (**Appendix A Table 1**).

Regulation of Dietary Supplements in the United States

In October 1994, the U.S. Government passed the Dietary Supplement Health and Education Act (DSHEA). This act amended the Federal Food, Drug, and Cosmetic Act and significantly changed the regulation of dietary supplements in the United States. This act also created a new regulatory framework for establishing the safety and labeling of dietary supplements. Before this act, dietary supplements were subject to the same regulatory requirements as other foods. Under DSHEA, however, the manufacturers or distributors of dietary supplements became responsible for determining the safety of their dietary supplements. Additionally, this act does not compel manufacturers to provide the U.S. Food and Drug Administration (FDA) with the evidence they rely on to substantiate safety or effectiveness before or after they market their products. Likewise, the FDA does not need to approve dietary supplements before marketing. Manufacturers are required, however, to show evidence that any representations or claims about the dietary supplement are not false or misleading. After a supplement reaches market, the FDA is responsible for regulating and taking action against any unsafe dietary supplement. As such, the manufacturer, packer, or distributor is required to submit to the FDA all serious adverse event reports associated with use of the dietary supplement in the United States. Despite this responsibility, however, there is no formal postmarketing surveillance of supplements. As a result, consumers and health care providers are responsible for reporting serious adverse events to the manufacturer or FDA.

Use of Vitamin and Mineral Supplements in the United States

Vitamin and mineral supplements are the most commonly used dietary supplements in the United States[9] and are available in numerous forms (e.g., individual vitamins, minerals, and multivitamin combinations). According to the National Health and Nutrition Examination Survey III, nearly half of the U.S. population (44% of men, 53% of women) reported using a dietary supplement. Multivitamin supplements are the most common (**Table 2**),[10] and supplement use has also increased over time.[11] In 2010, vitamins accounted for 34 percent of the $28.1 billion in annual sales of dietary supplement in the United States and minerals accounted for 8 percent.[12]

Individuals primarily use vitamin and mineral supplements to promote health and/or to prevent and mitigate disease. The National Family Opinion for the Natural Marketing Institute surveyed a representative sample of U.S. heads of households (n=2,002) regarding their motivations for using supplements.[13] This survey found that over 65 percent of respondents reported they used vitamin or mineral supplements to improve health and wellness. In addition, nearly 50 percent of respondents felt that dietary supplements helped prevent and treat cancer and heart disease. In a series of surveys of health care providers (Healthcare Professionals [HCP] Impact Study), 57 to 96 percent of respondents said they personally used dietary supplements at least occasionally, primarily for health and wellbeing.[14-16]

Current Clinical Practice in the United States

In the HCP Impact Study, 72 percent of physicians (n=900), 89 percent of nurses (n=277), and 97 percent of registered dietitians (n=300) surveyed recommended dietary supplements to patients for their overall health and wellness.[14,16] Among 300 cardiologists responding to the same 2008 survey, 55 percent of those who recommended using dietary supplements reported heart health as the primary reason for the recommendation to their patients.[15] Several professional organizations and Federal agencies have made recommendations about using multivitamin supplements to prevent chronic disease (**Table 3**). These groups concluded that there is insufficient evidence to make a recommendation for the use of dietary supplements in the prevention of chronic disease in the general population. They advise patients to obtain essential nutrients through diet.

Prevalence and Burden of CVD and Cancer in the United States

Incidence and Mortality

Over 1.2 million people experience a first or recurrent coronary event and nearly 800,000 have a stroke each year in the United States (**Table 4**).[17] CVD is increasingly affecting the elderly (age 65 years and older) and affects more men than women.[17] Additionally, the prevalence of coronary heart disease is greatest among American Indians/Native Americans (11.6%), followed by blacks (6.5%), Hispanics (6.1%), and whites (5.8%).[18] Asians and Pacific Islanders have the lowest prevalence (3.9%).[18]

Heart disease is the leading cause of death in the United States across both sexes and all races and ethnicities (**Table 5**).[19] In 2009, CVD (i.e., coronary heart disease, hypertensive heart disease, heart failure, and stroke) accounted for about one in every three deaths in the United States (age-adjusted mortality rate, 243.9 per 100,000).[17] Over one third (34%) of CVD deaths occurred in people younger than age 75 years.[17] Coronary heart disease (myocardial infarction [MI], angina, and sudden death) accounted for about half of CVD deaths; stroke accounted for 16 percent of CVD deaths.[17] In 2009, men were more likely to die from CVD than women (age-adjusted mortality rate, 287.2 per 100,000 men vs. 196.1 per 100,000 women).[17] These mortality rates were higher among blacks in both sexes than whites. American Indian/Alaskan Natives and Asian/Pacific Islanders had lower rates among both sexes.

In 2012, over 1.6 million individuals were diagnosed with cancer in the United States.[20] The annual age-adjusted incidence rate for any cancer was 465.2 per 100,000 individuals, with men about 1.3 times more likely to be diagnosed with cancer than women. The median age at diagnosis was 66 years. **Table 6** gives the incidence of the major types of cancer stratified by sex and race/ethnicity, derived from the National Cancer Institute Surveillance Epidemiology and End Results Program. Among men, cancer rates are highest in black males. These rates are primarily driven by high prostate cancer incidence rates. Black men also have the highest incidence of lung cancer compared with other sex-race/ethnicity groups. Cancer rates are lowest in Asian/Pacific Islander women (a grouping that likely hides considerable heterogeneity). Among women, whites have the highest overall incidence of cancer, mainly due to relatively high rates of breast cancer. Cancer rates are also high in black women. Black women have a breast cancer incidence only slightly lower than that of white women, and black women have the highest rates of colorectal cancer among women.[20]

In 2009, cancer was the second leading cause of death in the United States, and 570,000 cancer deaths were expected in 2012.[19,20] The overall age-adjusted mortality rate for any cancer was 178.7 per 100,000 individuals, with a median age at death of 72 years. These rates differed by sex, and men were more likely to die from cancer than women (219.4 vs. 151.1 per 100,000). Prostate cancer in men and breast cancer in women are the main contributors to cancer mortality.

Colorectal cancer and lung cancer are also contributors in both sexes (**Table 7**). Black men and women have the highest total cancer mortality and the highest mortality rates for all the major cancer sites.[20] Prostate cancer mortality in black men is more than twice that in other race/ethnic groups.[20]

Traditional Risk Factors and Common Pathologic Mechanisms for CVD and Cancer

The risk factors for CVD are quite well-established and include age, sex, blood pressure, smoking status, and blood cholesterol level. The effects of age and sex are interrelated. This is evidenced by the fact that women generally develop CVD when they are about 10 years older than men. Randomized, controlled trials (RCTs) have definitively established the causal relationship between elevated blood pressure and cholesterol levels and CVD. There are many other factors that affect CVD risk, including genetic variation. The major risk factors of elevated blood pressure, abnormal lipid levels, and smoking, plus other lifestyle factors (diabetes; obesity; consumption of fruits, vegetables, sodium, and alcohol; psychosocial factors; and regular physical activity) account for about 90 percent of the variance in CVD rates worldwide.[21] Cancer risk is considerably more complex because of the varied nature of cancers and because both environmental factors and genetics are critically involved. Despite the differences in their clinical manifestations, CVD and cancer share several risk and etiologic factors. Cigarette smoking, poor nutrition, physical inactivity, and obesity are associated with both CVD and many cancers (particularly breast and colorectal). Inflammation and oxidative stress, both prime targets of vitamin and mineral supplements, appear to account for at least part of this overlap. Cigarette smoke contains many oxidative compounds, while dietary fruits and vegetables contain high amounts of antioxidant compounds, and regular physical activity is associated with lower levels of inflammatory markers.[22] Inflammation and high oxidative potential produce arterial wall damage and exacerbate the impact of hypertension and dyslipidemia.[23] The most atherogenic forms of low-density lipoprotein (LDL) are highly susceptible to oxidation, and only oxidized LDL particles stimulate atherosclerosis.[24] Oxidative damage to DNA causes formation of multiple aberrations, including DNA adducts, methylation, single strand breaks, and genomic instability, that likely lead to mutagenesis and oncogenesis.[25]

Another possible common pathway for CVD and cancer etiology is methionine metabolism. Methionine is a sulfur-containing amino acid derived from dietary sources (particularly animal protein) and intracellular turnover of proteins. Methionine metabolism results in the generation of S-adenosylmethionine, an important methyl donor to RNA, DNA, proteins, and other compounds. Methylation may interfere with tumor suppressor genes and produce chromosomal aberrations that contribute to oncogenesis.[26,27] The methionine cycle also includes homocysteine, a cytotoxic compound that is an independent risk factor for CVD.[28] Interestingly, the conversion of homocysteine to methionine is the major route for eliminating the former compound from cardiovascular cells and is dependent on B vitamins, including, but not limited to, B_{12} and folate.

Role of Vitamins and Minerals in the Prevention of CVD and Cancer

The principal rationale for advocating multivitamin supplementation in both CVD and cancer prevention is the overlap of risk factors, particularly inflammation, oxidative stress, and methionine metabolism. This is important given that several dietary supplements are known to have antioxidant and anti-inflammatory effects or influence methionine metabolism. This has served as the rationale for proposing dietary supplements as an effective means to prevent both CVD and cancer.

Oxidative damage by free radicals and other reactive species is ubiquitous and there are numerous, interacting biochemical mechanisms by which vitamins and/or minerals might protect against these effects, thus reducing both CVD and cancer risk. Fat-soluble antioxidant vitamins such as vitamin E circulate principally in lipoproteins, especially LDLs. As noted above, oxidized LDL is highly atherogenic and vitamin E protects against this oxidation. To maintain vitamin E in its antioxidant or reduced state, however, circulating, water-soluble antioxidants such as vitamin C are required. Natural, enzymatic antioxidants (e.g., superoxide dismutase, glutathione peroxidase) catalyze the reactions that suppress free radicals and peroxide and contain copper, zinc, and manganese as integral parts of their structure, providing a rationale for supplementing with minerals.

Several B vitamins (folate, B_6, and B_{12}) are important in homocysteine metabolism. This is important given that about half of the homocysteine generated in a typical diet is metabolized through transsulfuration, which does not generate methionine and is dependent on B_6. The other half of this homocysteine is remethylated to methionine through reactions that require folate and B_{12} as cofactors. As methyl donors, these vitamins are also essential for normal nucleotide and DNA synthesis and repair. High doses of these vitamins could have negative consequences, however, as hypermethylation may contribute to oncogenesis. In addition, numerous clinical trials conducted over the past decade have failed to show benefit of high-dose folic acid supplementation despite favorable effects on serum homocysteine levels.[29] Some observers posit that these overall negative results could be hiding important subgroup differences,[30] including baseline levels of B vitamins and renal function. These issues illustrate the complexities created by the interrelationships of genetics, diet, and supplementation.

Vitamin E (gamma-tocopherol), zinc, and vitamin A are thought to inhibit inflammation, another presumed protective mechanism provided by vitamins and minerals. In addition, other effects of vitamins may be relevant to other chronic diseases, such as enhanced immunity (vitamins A, C, and E and zinc and calcium) or stimulation of collagen synthesis (vitamin C). The implications of these effects for CVD and cancer, however, remain uncertain. Other effects, such as regulation of cell differentiation, proliferation, and apoptosis may be related to these diseases. Research has also suggested that vitamins A, C, and D and alpha-tocopherol inhibit angiogenesis, which might help prevent cancer. This effect, however, would likely exacerbate vascular disease.[31-36]

Normal human exposure to vitamins and minerals is through diet (any intake of food), which includes a vast array of known and unknown micronutrients that interact in complex ways with each other and with macronutrients, such as fiber and fatty acids. This is complicated further by the fact that individuals may absorb and metabolize food in ways that influence the effects of these nutrients. As such, even the most complex multivitamin cannot hope to mimic the content of a healthful diet that includes a wide variety of unprocessed foods. Additionally, the components of single vitamin or multivitamin supplements may vary substantially from what is found in whole foods, which could alter biological impact. Vitamin E, for example, exists in eight chemical forms in food, with gamma-tocopherol being the most abundant form in the U.S. diet (**Appendix A Table 1**). However, vitamin E supplements generally contain alpha-tocopherol, which is also abundant in the diet but can act as a pro-oxidant under some circumstances. Whether or not this pro-oxidant effect of alpha-tocopherol is important in vivo or affects the stability or potency of other nutrients in a combined pill is unknown, but it illustrates the complexity of vitamin supplementation. The importance of a supplement's chemical form and potential vitamin-vitamin interaction can be exponentially expanded when we consider its potential interactions with other nutrients, supplements, and medications.

For these reasons, the use of vitamin and mineral supplements cannot be recommended based solely on mechanistic studies. Similarly, multiple biases and confounding by unmeasured covariates can affect the results of cohort (longitudinal) studies. These limitations diminish the ability of cohort studies to establish a causal link. As such, RCTs are essential to proving benefit and detecting harm. Unfortunately, the number of trials available for multiple and single vitamins is quite small considering the widespread use of these agents. This is partly due to the special regulatory environment for supplements and the lack of incentive for manufacturers to conduct randomized trials.

Previous USPSTF Recommendation

In 2003, the USPSTF concluded that the current evidence was insufficient to assess the balance of benefits and harms of the use of supplements of vitamins A, C, or E; multivitamins with folic acid; or antioxidant combinations for the prevention of cancer or CVD in asymptomatic adults (I statement). This review found poor-quality evidence to determine if vitamins reduce the risk for CVD or cancer, and available RCTs were inadequate or conflicting. Based on this review, the USPSTF recommended against the use of beta-carotene supplements, either alone or in combination, for the prevention of cancer or CVD in asymptomatic adults (D recommendation). This recommendation was based on good-quality evidence that beta-carotene had no benefit in the prevention of CVD and cancer and actually might cause harm in some adult populations (i.e., an increased risk of lung cancer in heavy smokers).[1]

Chapter 2. Methods

AHRQ commissioned this evidence review on the use of multivitamins for the primary prevention of cancer and CVD in the general population to assist the USPSTF in updating its 2003 recommendation on routine vitamin supplementation. Our review is similar in scope to the three 2003 evidence reviews[37-39] the USPSTF used to develop its previous recommendation statement.[1] These reviews, however, included a limited number of individual and combination vitamins and minerals (vitamins A, E, and C, "antioxidant combinations," and "multivitamin preparations") compared with our review, which includes additional supplements (e.g., calcium, vitamin D, folic acid). In addition, the previous reviews included any primary or secondary prevention study of vitamins or minerals that reported on the incidence or mortality of cancer[38] or CVD,[37] whereas our review focused on primary prevention.

In 2006, Huang and colleagues conducted a comprehensive and good-quality systematic review for a National Institute of Health State-of-the-Science Conference on the efficacy and safety of multivitamin and mineral supplement use to prevent cancer and chronic disease in adults.[40] This review focused on the prevention of all chronic conditions, including CVD and cancer. We used this existing review as the foundation for our current review.

Key Questions and Analytic Framework

We developed an analytic framework (**Figure 1**) and four Key Questions (KQs) to guide our literature searches in consultation with members from the USPSTF. This review addressed the following KQs:

1. What is the efficacy of multivitamin supplement use on health outcomes in the general adult population?
2. What is known about the safety of multivitamin supplement use in the general adult population?
3. What is the efficacy of supplementation with single nutrients or functionally related nutrient pairs on health outcomes in the general adult population?
4. What is known about the safety of single nutrient use in the general adult population?

Data Sources and Searches

We performed comprehensive literature searches in the following databases: MEDLINE, EMBASE, Cochrane Database of Systematic Reviews, Database of Abstracts of Reviews of Effects, and Cochrane Central Register of Controlled Trials from 2005 through January 29, 2013 to identify studies published since the 2006 review by Huang and colleagues. We worked with an expert library scientist to develop comprehensive literature search strategies (**Appendix B**). We limited all searches to articles published in the English language. The literature search results were managed using version 12.0 of Reference Manager (Thomson Reuters, New York, NY).

We reviewed the reference lists of included studies and relevant systematic reviews and meta-analyses to identify relevant articles that were published before the timeframe of our literature searches or were not identified by our searches to ensure our retrieval strategy was comprehensive. We obtained references from outside experts and bibliographies of other relevant sources (e.g., dietary guidelines). We also searched Federal agency trial registries for ongoing and/or unpublished trials (**Appendix C**). We conducted a search of the grey literature that included summary reports from the Center for Food Safety and Nutrition Adverse Events Reporting System. We also evaluated all studies included and excluded in the four previous reviews against the inclusion and exclusion criteria for the current review.[37-40] As a result, we included 10 studies from the previous reviews (published in 30 articles). We also conducted a supplementary search examining dietary supplements to prevent diabetes mellitus.

For KQs 1 and 3 (efficacy), we restricted the searches to include only RCTs, systematic reviews, and meta-analyses. For KQs 2 and 4 (safety), we expanded our searches to include observational studies (e.g., cohort or registry-based studies) and postmarketing surveillance data.

Study Selection

Two reviewers independently reviewed the titles and abstracts of all identified articles against inclusion and exclusion criteria for design, population, intervention, and outcomes (**Appendix B Table 1**). Two reviewers independently evaluated the full-text article(s) of all potentially included studies against the complete inclusion and exclusion criteria (**Appendix B Table 1**). We resolved disagreements in the abstract and/or full-text review through discussion and consultation with a third reviewer.

For efficacy (KQs 1 and 3), we included primary prevention trials (i.e., prevention of development of disease in a population or individual who is well and does not have the disease in question)[41] that addressed the outcomes of interest to the USPSTF. These outcomes included any CVD incidence (e.g., coronary heart disease, ischemic heart disease, coronary artery disease, atherosclerotic heart disease, atherosclerosis, and diabetes), cardiomyopathy, angina pectoris (i.e., chest pain), MI, stroke (both ischemic and hemorrhagic and cerebrovascular accidents), heart failure and related mortality, cancer incidence and related mortality, and all-cause mortality. We included only trials that addressed these as a priori outcomes and included a general population not selected due to poor nutrition. Because of the generally limited number of primary prevention trials, we also included trials that evaluated secondary prevention (i.e., prevention of disease in individuals with a previous diagnosis or serious risk factors) if the study also hypothesized effects on other outcomes. For example, the Skin Cancer Prevention Study (SCPS), the Retinoid Skin Cancer Prevention trials (Skin Cancer Prevention-Actinic Keratoses [SKICAP-AK] and Skin Cancer Prevention-SCC/BCC [SKICAP-S/B]), and the Nambour Skin Cancer and Actinic Eye Disease Prevention trial were designed to prevent skin cancer in patients with a prior history of basal cell carcinoma (BCC) and/or squamous cell carcinoma (SCC) of the skin with a vitamin or mineral supplement. We included these trials because they also hypothesized that supplementation might impact other cancers and mortality. For these studies, we only considered nonskin cancer and only used all-cause mortality and/or harms data (if reported) in our synthesis. We also excluded tertiary prevention trials (i.e., prevention of complications or recurrence of a disease in a symptomatic person who has been diagnosed with the disease). For mortality, we also included studies designed to prevent other diseases if they reported all-cause mortality data as a primary aim. We did not include any reported CVD or cancer outcomes for studies whose primary aim was not to prevent these two conditions. For harms, we included any trial that reported on adverse events, regardless of its aim.

We included studies that examined the efficacy of multivitamins (KQs 1 and 2); calcium; folic acid; vitamins B_1, B_2, B_6, B_{12}, E, C, A, and D; iron; zinc; magnesium; niacin; calcium/magnesium; calcium/vitamin D; folic acid/vitamin B_{12}; and folic acid/vitamin B_6 (KQ 3). For examination of safety (KQ 4), we specifically focused on the following supplements that had hypothesized harms: calcium; folic acid; vitamin D; calcium/vitamin D, E, and A; iron; selenium; and beta-carotene.

We only included studies that tested supplements at doses lower than their tolerable upper intake level. As such, we excluded studies evaluating high-dose vitamin therapy. This decision reflects our focus on recommendations for preventive vitamin and mineral supplementation, as opposed to therapeutic supplementation. **Appendix A Table 1** lists the RDA and upper intake levels for the micronutrients we included in the review.

For KQs 1 and 3, we selected RCTs in community-dwelling adults (age 18 years or older) who did not have chronic disease or nutritional deficiencies. We included populations with hypertension and/or hypercholesterolemia as long as they did not have known CVD (e.g., coronary, cerebrovascular, or peripheral artery disease) or diabetes. We excluded studies in which 10 percent or more of participants had active/current CVD, diabetes mellitus, or cancer, as we did not want a significant proportion of the study population to have chronic diseases and to reduce any confounders.

For KQs 2 and 4, we selected RCTs or longitudinal observational studies (e.g., prospective cohort studies) in community-dwelling adults who were without chronic disease or nutritional deficiencies. We included observational studies to increase the likelihood of detecting harms that are rare or that develop only after long time periods.[42] We focused on important harms by including only those adverse events that were reported in more than 5 percent of the study population or met the definition of serious events used by the study investigators and that occurred at a significantly higher rate in the intervention group(s). Furthermore, we did not include observational study data on the main outcomes being examined—CVD, cancer, and all-cause mortality—but rather included only RCT data for these outcomes, whether beneficial or (paradoxically) harmful.

We only included studies that were conducted in countries the Human Development Index classifies as "very high" to avoid the possibility of widespread nutritional deficiencies in other countries.[43] Supplementation in a nutrient-deficient population would be considered treatment of a disorder, and therefore was excluded.

Quality Assessment

Two reviewers independently assessed the methodological quality of each study using predefined criteria developed by the USPSTF[44] and supplemented with the National Institute for Health and Clinical Excellence methodology checklists for observational studies (**Appendix B**

Table 2).[45] We resolved disagreements in quality through discussion. We assigned each study a final quality rating of good, fair, or poor.

Good-quality RCTs were those with adequate randomization procedures and allocation concealment, blinded outcome assessment, reliable outcome measures, similar groups at baseline (i.e., little to no statistically significant differences between groups in baseline demographics and characteristics), low attrition (≥90% of participants had followup data, with <10 percentage-point difference in loss to followup between groups), and those that used conservative data-substitution methods if missing data were inferred. Trials were downgraded to fair quality if they did not meet the majority of the good-quality criteria. We rated trials as poor quality if attrition was greater than 40 percent or differed between groups by 20 percentage points, or if there were any other important "fatal" flaws that two independent investigators agreed seriously affected internal validity. Poor-quality studies were excluded from the review (**Appendix D**).

Good-quality observational studies had an unbiased selection of the nonexposed cohort, adequate ascertainment of exposure, addressed a population without the outcome of interest at the beginning of the study, reliable outcome measures, blinded assessment, low attrition, adjustment for potential confounders, and no other important threats to internal validity. Observational studies were downgraded to fair quality if they were unable to meet the majority of good-quality criteria. Poor-quality observational studies had multiple threats to internal validity and were excluded from the review.

Data Extraction

One reviewer abstracted data from all included studies rated as fair- or good-quality into a standard evidence table and a second reviewer checked the data for accuracy. We abstracted population characteristics (e.g., baseline demographics, body mass index, concurrent conditions, family history of cancer or CVD, smoking status, alcohol use, physical activity, and prior supplement use), study design (e.g., recruitment procedures, inclusion/exclusion criteria, followup, and population adherence), and intervention characteristics (e.g., supplements, chemical form, dose, frequency, duration of use, and timing of use), as well as health outcomes.

We abstracted health outcomes that included the number of participants experiencing an event and incidence rates. For cancer outcomes, we abstracted any data on solid or hematologic malignancies and related deaths; we did not abstract data on precancerous lesions (e.g., cervical intraepithelial neoplasia). For cardiovascular health outcomes, we abstracted any CVD (e.g., coronary heart disease, ischemic heart disease, coronary artery disease, atherosclerotic heart disease, atherosclerosis, and diabetes), cardiomyopathy, angina pectoris (i.e., chest pain), MI, stroke (both ischemic and hemorrhagic and cerebrovascular accidents), heart failure, and related deaths. We did not abstract cardiovascular symptoms, such as palpitations and arrhythmias, or risk factors (e.g., blood pressure, lipid levels). For all-cause mortality, we abstracted all-cause mortality rates. For adverse events, as mentioned previously, we abstracted only those events that were reported in more than 5 percent of participants, if there was a significant difference among the interventions groups, and if they were serious adverse events as defined by the study.

Data Synthesis and Analysis

We synthesized the results of the included studies of the four KQs in related pairs (i.e., KQs 1 and 2 for multivitamin supplements, KQs 3 and 4 for single and paired supplements). For KQs 3 and 4, the results are grouped by single supplement: beta-carotene, vitamin E, selenium, vitamin A, vitamin C, folic acid, vitamin D, and calcium. Paired or combination supplements are discussed under each individual supplement (e.g., beta-carotene in combination with vitamin A is discussed under two sections: beta-carotene and vitamin A), as included studies reported minimal interaction effects with combination supplements. Vitamin D and calcium combination supplements were discussed separately from calcium alone and vitamin D alone.

We created summary evidence tables for each supplement showing the main outcomes (i.e., CVD incidence, cancer incidence, mortality, and harms) along with important population characteristics and study design features. We critically examined the population characteristics and design features to identify the range of results and potential associations with heterogeneity of treatment effects across studies. Other study design and baseline demographics are provided in **Appendix E**.

For each supplement, we created results tables for CVD (CVD incidence and cardiovascular-related deaths), cancer (any, the four major site-specific cancers [lung, colorectal, prostate, breast], and cancer-related deaths), and all-cause mortality. Other cancers were briefly discussed if there were statistically significant differences between groups within a particular study or if there were differences across studies; otherwise, we indicated that there was no statistically significant effect on other cancers.

The results tables include the number of participants experiencing an event and study-reported relative risks (RRs), hazard ratios (HRs), odds ratios (ORs), confidence intervals (CIs), and p-values. Most studies reported adjusted outcome measures; therefore, we did not calculate unadjusted risk ratios. We examined the CIs and/or p-values to determine if an estimate reached statistical significance. We examined these estimates to determine if a supplement had a statistically significant effect on an outcome (beneficial or harmful) within a specific trial and across trials examining the same supplement. We noted any patterns across studies and explained any clinical heterogeneity across trials that might clarify any differences in results. None of the included studies adjusted the significance level for testing of multiple outcomes (e.g., overall cancer plus several site-specific cancers); we focused on the main outcomes of the trials (all CVD, all cancer, all-cause mortality), limiting the impact of multiple testing. We include data on the components of these main outcomes, but the statistical comparisons should not be interpreted as hypothesis tests.

Eight of the included RCTs used factorial designs (usually 2x2, but also including more arms). These studies appropriately report the results for each arm as designed, thus comparing all participants who received one of the interventions with all those who did not, ignoring the assignments to the other intervention in the two groups. Analysis of factorial studies should include a formal test for interaction between the components, since if such interaction is present, the main effects cannot be interpreted and analysis should be conducted for the separate arms. Most of the factorial studies did provide a test for interaction between the interventions and found none, although the power of the studies to detect an interaction was not presented. Two studies did report comparisons across individual cells, generally the cell receiving only one supplement with the cell receiving only placebo. We ignored these analyses in the synthesis since they are essentially post hoc and are not fully valid in the absence of an interaction. Furthermore, these analyses did not produce different results from the factorial analyses. The results by individual arm for these studies are provided in **Appendix F Tables 1–6**, **Appendix F Figures 1** and **2**.

We found few trials examining the use of a multivitamin supplement in the prevention of CVD and cancer; three RCTs addressed KQ 1 (benefits of multivitamin supplement use) and five studies addressed KQ 2 (harms of multivitamin supplement use). We identified a substantial body of evidence addressing the benefits (KQ 3) and harms (KQ 4) of single or functionally related pairs; there were very few trials included per supplement. We examined the evidence qualitatively and, when appropriate, quantitatively. We conducted meta-analyses to estimate the effect size of supplementation on CVD incidence, cancer incidence, and all-cause mortality for the longest followup time point (**Figures 2–4**). Additional forest plots for site-specific cancers (lung, colorectal, prostate, and breast only), MI, strokes, and CVD-related and cancer-related deaths are available in **Appendix G Figures 1–12**.

We used Stata 11.2 (StataCorp LP, College State, TX) for all meta-analyses, entering the number of events and nonevents using the metan procedure.[46] Since most of the included outcomes were relatively rare, to avoid bias associated with rare events we used either Peto's OR method (when events typically occurred in <1% of participants) or a fixed effects risk ratio model using the Mantel-Haenszel method (when events typically occurred in 1% to 10% of participants).[47] When events were more common (>10% of participants), we conducted random effects analyses of risk ratios using the DerSimonian and Laird method.[48] We examined the I^2 statistic as a measure of statistical heterogeneity. We had too few trials to examine funnel plots for small-study effects. For most supplements, however, there were too few studies reporting similar outcomes in similar individuals for the pooled data to be interpretable; thus, for most supplements, the pooled analysis serves mainly to illustrate the results across the available trials that are discussed qualitatively. The overall pooled, unadjusted RR should not be overinterpreted due to the aforementioned clinical heterogeneity. In addition, the results from our meta-analysis may differ from those reported in original trials, as we used raw data and calculated unadjusted RRs and ORs. Throughout the report, we reference adjusted RRs, HRs, and ORs as reported in trials, unless we discuss pooled results.

USPSTF Involvement

This research was funded by AHRQ under a contract to support the work of the USPSTF. We consulted with four USPSTF liaisons at key points in the review, particularly in the development of the KQs, analytic framework, and the inclusion and exclusion criteria, as well as finalizing the evidence synthesis. An AHRQ Medical Officer provided oversight of the project, reviewed the draft report, and assisted in the external review of the report. AHRQ had no role in the study selection, quality assessment, or evidence synthesis.

Chapter 3. Results

Literature Search

Our literature search yielded 12,766 unique citations. From these, we provisionally accepted 277 articles for review based on titles and abstracts (**Appendix B Figure 1**). After screening the full-text articles, we judged 26 studies (103 articles) to have met the inclusion criteria. We excluded the remaining 174 full-text articles (**Appendix D**).

KQ 1. What Is the Efficacy of Multivitamin Supplement Use on Health Outcomes in the General Adult Population?

KQ 2. What Is Known About the Safety of Multivitamin Supplement Use in the General Adult Population?

Summary of Results

We identified four good-quality RCTs (n=28,607)[49-52] and one good-quality cohort study (n=72,337)[53] that evaluated the health effects of a multivitamin supplement (**Table 8**; **Appendix E Tables 1** and **2**); studies varied in which nutrients were included in the multivitamin formulation and their dosages (**Table 9**), as well as in the duration of supplement use and outcomes evaluated. No impact on all-cause mortality was found in any of the three RCTS reporting this outcome: the Supplementation in Vitamins and Mineral Antioxidants Study (SU.VI.MAX),[49] the Physician's Health Study II (PHS-II),[50] or the Roche European American Cataract Trial (REACT).[51] In REACT, which included 297 elderly European men and women, there were more deaths reported in the intervention group (n=9) than in the control group (n=3) after 3 years, but this difference was not statistically significant (p=0.07). When these data were pooled, there was no effect on all-cause mortality (unadjusted RR, 0.95 [95% CI, 0.81 to 1.11]), even in a sensitivity analysis with REACT removed (unadjusted RR, 0.95 [95% CI, 0.89 to 1.01]; data not shown).

In the two RCTs reporting CVD and cancer outcomes (SU.VI.MAX and PHS-II), multivitamins had no impact on most types of fatal and nonfatal CVD events, and the small benefit for fatal MI with supplementation reported in one trial (PHS-II) could be a type I error due to multiple testing. In contrast, both trials suggested a small reduction in overall cancer incidence in men after 11.2 to 12.5 years of followup. The age-adjusted HR for total cancer was 0.92 (95% CI, 0.86 to 0.998) among 14,641 male physicians older than age 50 years taking Centrum Silver® (Pfizer, Kings Mountain, NC) after 11.2 years of followup.[50] In a general population of middle-aged adults (n=13,017), SU.VI.MAX indicated no impact on overall cancer from a five-component multivitamin formulation after an initial followup of 7.5 years and posttreatment followup of an additional 5 years.[54] However, based on a significant sex-by-treatment group interaction (p=0.02), a sex-specific subgroup analysis showed a protective effect on any cancer (RR, 0.69 [95% CI, 0.53 to 0.91]) among men, but not women.

No consistent evidence of harms from nutritional dosages of multivitamins emerged from four RCTs[50-52,55] and a cohort study (Nurses' Health Study [NHS]),[53] although the possible harms from supplementation reported in individual studies or in subgroup analyses (e.g., increased melanomas among women enrolled in SU.VI.MAX, trend toward increased death among the REACT antioxidant group) warrant additional research.

Study Details

SU.VI.MAX was a double-blind, placebo-controlled RCT designed to test the hypothesis that daily supplementation with antioxidant vitamins and minerals reduced the incidence of major health problems, particularly CVD and cancer.[54] SU.VI.MAX supplements used "nutritional" doses (one to three times the RDA) of vitamin C (120 mg), vitamin E (30 mg), and beta-carotene (6 mg), plus selenium (100 mcg) and zinc (20 mg). Randomization was stratified by sex and age, and baseline characteristics were balanced between groups. Adherence to the medication was high (>70%) and comparable in both groups. We rated the overall quality of the study as good.

SU.VI.MAX recruited a general adult population in France, including men ages 45 to 60 years and women ages 35 to 60 years who were basically healthy and not taking a supplement containing any of the study agents. Recruitment was through a national public media campaign in 1994; almost 80,000 people responded, of which 21,481 returned a questionnaire and 14,412 were eligible. The 13,017 participants randomized into the trial had a mean age of 49 years; 59 percent were women. SU.VI.MAX reported its primary outcomes at the end of the active intervention phase of the trial (7.5 years after randomization).[49] Although it no longer provided supplements, SU.VI.MAX reported primary outcomes again 5 years later (12.5 years after randomization).[56]

PHS-II was a randomized, double-blind, placebo-controlled trial testing the effects of a multivitamin on CVD and cancer. PHS-II employed a 2x2x2x2 factorial design to test the effects of vitamin E, vitamin C, and beta-carotene, as well as a multivitamin. Results from two other arms of this trial are included in KQs 2 and 4. PHS-II used a multivitamin widely marketed in the United States (Centrum Silver) that contained 32 ingredients. The full list of ingredients appears in **Table 9**. Except for vitamins E and B_{12}, the doses did not exceed the RDA.

PHS-II recruited in two phases. In the first, 18,763 men from PHS-I were invited to participate, of which 7,641 were eligible and willing and were randomized. In the second phase, 254,597 additional physicians were contacted, of which 42,165 completed a baseline questionnaire and 7,000 were randomized.[50] Randomization was concealed and stratified by 5-year age group, prior history of CVD or cancer, and previous assignment to beta-carotene (for PHS-I participants). Baseline characteristics were balanced. All participants were male physicians, with a mean age at baseline of 64 years. Followup was greater than 98 percent and self-reported adherence was above 70 percent through 8 years of followup and 67 percent at the end of the trial, without differences by group. We rated the overall quality of the study as good.

The other two multivitamin RCTs provided data on all-cause mortality and/or harms. REACT was a good-quality RCT that used a combination of three antioxidants (vitamin C [250 mg], vitamin E [200 mg], and beta-carotene [6 mg]) to prevent progression of early age-related cataracts in 297 men and women (mean age, 66.2 years).[51] Similarly, the study by Graat and colleagues was a small, good-quality RCT included for harms only. It evaluated the efficacy of a 26-component multivitamin supplement (components listed in **Table 9**) to reduce the incidence and severity of acute respiratory infections in older adults (n=652; mean age, 73.2 years).[52] It also included a vitamin E (200 mg) supplement in a 2x2 factorial design. A single good-quality prospective cohort study (NHS) among 72,337 postmenopausal registered nurses (mean age, 58.3 years) provided additional data regarding harms.[53] It evaluated the relationship of vitamin A intake in multivitamins and the risk of hip fractures.

CVD

Two trials (n=27,658) reported CVD outcomes (**Table 10**, **Figure 2**).[49,57] Primary cardiovascular outcomes reported in SU.VI.MAX (n=13,017) included major fatal and nonfatal ischemic cardiovascular events. Overall, there was no effect on ischemic CVD events after 7.5 years of supplementation; incidence was 2.1 percent in both arms (RR, 0.97 [95% CI, 0.77 to 1.20]). Although the RR was lower in men, it was not statistically significant, and the sex-by-group interaction was also not significant (p=0.44). The results after an additional 5 years of followup (without further provision of the vitamins) were almost identical (RR, 0.97 [95% CI, 0.80 to 1.17]). SU.VI.MAX did not report on the incidence of diabetes mellitus.

The primary CVD outcomes reported in PHS-II were any major cardiovascular event, including nonfatal MI, nonfatal stroke, and CVD mortality. PHS-II also found no effect on CVD after 11.2 years of followup, with 12 percent incidence of any CVD in both arms (HR, 1.01 [95% CI, 0.91 to 1.10]).[57] There were also no statistically significant differences between groups on the number of participants with an MI and stroke (any, ischemic, or hemorrhagic). There was also no statistically significant difference in the number of CVD-related deaths (HR, 0.95 [95% CI, 0.83 to 1.09]). The number of fatal MIs, however, was borderline statistically significant (p=0.048) in favor of the intervention. There was no adjustment, however, for multicomparisons.

Cancer

Two trials (n=27,658) reported cancer outcomes (**Table 11**, **Figure 3**).[49,50] The primary cancer outcome for SU.VI.MAX was incident cancer of any kind (except BCC of the skin). There was no significant difference between groups for overall cancer incidence (RR, 0.90 [95% CI, 0.76 to 1.06]). The results, however, differed by sex. A significant sex-by-group interaction was observed (p=0.02), with a protective effect of the multivitamin in men (p=0.008) but no effect in women (p=0.53). For men, the RR of any cancer was 0.69 (95% CI, 0.53 to 0.91), while for women, the RR was 1.04 (95% CI, 0.85 to 1.29). It is possible that effects were only seen in men in SU.VI.MAX because they were older than the women (mean age, 51.3 years in men vs. 46.6 years in women).

SU.VI.MAX also reported cancer incidence by cancer type. The multivitamin supplement had no effect on the incidence of hematological, thyroid, urinary tract, genital, respiratory tract, digestive tract, or oral cavity cancer, but tended toward very small, nonsignificant benefits for sex-specific cancers (i.e., prostate and breast) and possible sex-specific harms for skin cancer (data not shown).[49] After a followup of almost 9 years, prostate cancer occurred in 103 men: 49 in the supplement arm and 54 in the control group (p-value not significant).[55] Similarly, in women, there were five fewer breast cancers in the intervention group. After 7.5 years of followup, 157 skin cancers (i.e., melanoma at any stage, BCC, SCC, and other types of skin cancer) occurred overall; incidence was higher in women in the supplement arm (p=0.03), but not in men.[58] Most of this difference was due to higher rates of melanoma; the HR of melanoma for women taking supplementation was 4.31 (95% CI, 1.23 to 15.13). Deaths by cancer type were not reported.

PHS-II was designed to evaluate both overall and site-specific cancer rates in men (excluding nonmelanoma skin cancer [NMSC]).[50] After 11.2 years of followup, all-site cancer incidence was significantly reduced in the intervention group (17.6%) compared with the comparison group (18.8%) (HR, 0.92 [95% CI, 0.86 to 0.998]). Prostate, colorectal, lung, bladder, and pancreatic cancer, as well as lymphoma, leukemia, and melanoma incidence did not differ by intervention group in PHS-II. Cancer mortality did not differ by treatment, although it showed a trend favoring the intervention (HR, 0.88 [95% CI, 0.77 to 1.01]). There were no statistically significant effects on prostate, colorectal, lung, pancreatic, or other cancer (e.g., bladder) deaths; however, death rates for these cancers were uniformly lower in those taking the multivitamin supplement (**Table 11**).

When data from the two studies were pooled, the cancer incidence was significantly lower among men in the supplement groups (unadjusted RR, 0.93 [95% CI, 0.87 to 0.99]; I^2=0.0%; data not shown).

All-Cause Mortality

All-cause mortality (**Table 12**, **Figure 4**) was reported in three trials (n=27,955).[49-51] In SU.VI.MAX, overall mortality was lower in the supplement group, but the difference was not significant (RR, 0.77 [95% CI, 0.57 to 1.00]) after 7.5 years of followup. Mortality was significantly lower in men (RR, 0.63 [95% CI, 0.42 to 0.93]) but not in women (RR, 1.03 [95% CI, 0.64 to 1.63]). The sex-by-group interaction, however, was not significant (p=0.11).[49] The mortality rate was higher in PHS-II participants, who were much older, but the RR reduction was much smaller than for men in SU.VI.MAX (HR, 0.94 vs. RR, 0.63, respectively) and was not statistically significant (p=0.13) (note that the followup time was shorter in SU.VI.MAX). When data from the two studies were pooled, multivitamins did not have a statistically significant effect on all-cause mortality in men (RR, 0.94 [95% CI, 0.88 to 1.01]; I^2=37.9%; data not shown). There were only 12 deaths in REACT (n=297).[51] Nine deaths occurred in the treatment group and three in the control group (p=0.07), but these data are likely unreliable given the small number of deaths. When data from the three studies were pooled (**Figure 4**), there was no statistically significant effect on all-cause mortality with multivitamin supplementation (unadjusted RR, 0.95 [95% CI, 0.80 to 1.11]; I^2=42.5%), even with a sensitivity analysis removing REACT (unadjusted RR, 0.95 [95% CI, 0.89 to 1.01]; data not shown).

Harms

Four good-quality RCTs (n=28,607)[50-52,55] and one good-quality prospective cohort study (n=72,337)[53] reported on harms (**Appendix E Tables 1** and **2**). NHS examined the associations between hip fractures and multivitamin intake in postmenopausal women (aiming to examine the influence of the vitamin A component specifically).[53] This cohort study found a statistically significant increase in hip fractures among current multivitamin users compared with nonusers (RR, 1.32 [95% CI, 1.04 to 1.67]) and a nonsignificant increased risk among former users (RR, 1.25 [95% CI, 0.97 to 1.61]).

REACT reported that hypercarotenemia (yellowing of the skin) developed in six patients (presumably in the treatment arm).[51] Other side effects and intercurrent illnesses did not differ by treatment group and were not considered serious; no further details were provided. SU.VI.MAX reported minor side effects in less than 10 participants taking the multivitamin supplement, and none withdrew due to these side effects (no further details were provided).[55] PHS-II found no significant effects on gastrointestinal tract symptoms (e.g., peptic ulcer, constipation, gastritis, and nausea), fatigue, drowsiness, skin discoloration, or migraine.[50] Multivitamin supplement users were more likely to have rashes than the placebo group (p=0.03). PHS-II found mixed results for bleeding events, with significantly more cases of hematuria (p=0.02) and epistaxis (p=0.01) in the multivitamin group than the placebo group, but no difference in the number of participants who easily bruised or other bleeding events (p=0.77).[50]

The study by Graat and colleagues found no difference between groups in the incidence or severity of acute respiratory tract infection or in total illness duration, number of symptoms, number of fevers, number of participants with restriction to activity, or episode-related medication use, suggesting neither harm nor benefit for respiratory-related outcomes in older adults with multivitamin supplementation.[52]

KQ 3. What Is the Efficacy of Supplementation With Single Nutrients or Functionally Related Nutrient Pairs on Health Outcomes in the General Adult Population?

KQ 4. What Is Known About the Safety of Single Nutrient Use in the General Adult Population?

The third and fourth KQs for this review concerned single supplements and various pairs of supplements. We found no trials that reported incidence of CVD or cancer or all-cause mortality for four B vitamins (1, 2, 6, or 12), iron, zinc, magnesium, niacin, calcium/magnesium, folic acid/vitamin B_{12}, or folic acid/vitamin B_6. Overall, the available studies for beta-carotene; vitamins A, C, D, and E; selenium; folic acid; calcium; and some combinations found no evidence for a benefit of the supplement on CVD, cancer, or all-cause mortality. Instead, two studies using beta-carotene for those at high risk for lung cancer (i.e., smokers and/or asbestos-exposed workers) found that participants in the supplement groups were at a significantly higher risk of developing or dying from lung cancer.[59,60]

Beta-Carotene

Summary of Results

Six good-quality RCTs (n=112,820) examined beta-carotene supplementation alone or in combination with another study supplement, such as vitamin E or A (**Table 13**).[59-64] No effects were seen on CVD outcomes or on overall cancer incidence, but there was an increase in lung cancer incidence and mortality and in all-cause mortality in two trials of participants at high risk for lung cancer at baseline (i.e., smokers and/or asbestos-exposed workers).[59] One of these trials, which examined beta-carotene in combination with vitamin A, terminated early due to the increase in risk.[60] Yellowing of the skin was the most frequently reported adverse effect with beta-carotene supplementation.

Study Details

We identified six RCTs (n=112,820) examining the efficacy and safety of beta-carotene supplementation (**Appendix E Tables 1** and **2**): the Alpha-Tocopherol Beta-Carotene Cancer Prevention (ATBC) trial,[59] PHS-I,[61] the Women's Health Study (WHS),[62] SCPS,[63] the Nambour Skin Cancer Prevention Study (NSCPS),[64] and the Carotene and Retinol Efficacy Trial (CARET).[60] While two RCTs included for efficacy (SCPS and NSCPS) reported incidence of skin cancer, these trials were designed to examine the effectiveness of beta-carotene supplementation on the secondary prevention of skin cancer (i.e., prevention of new skin cancer in patients with BCC and/or SCC); thus, we only considered their mortality outcomes.[63,64]

The six RCTs examining the efficacy and/or safety of beta-carotene were all double-blind, placebo-controlled trials. Three were 2x2 factorial-designed trials randomizing participants to beta-carotene or another intervention (daily sunscreen,[64] vitamin E,[59] or aspirin[61]) and one was a 2x2x2 factorial-designed trial randomizing participants to beta-carotene, vitamin E, or aspirin.[62] One study randomized participants to a combination supplement of beta-carotene and vitamin A.[60] The doses ranged from 30 mg daily[60,64] to 50 mg daily[59,63] or every other day;[61,62] all other supplements (e.g., vitamins E, A) were within the DRI as set forth by the Food and Nutrition Board (**Appendix A Table 1**).

Two trials included only men, one included only women, and the others included both sexes. The ATBC trial was conducted among 29,133 male smokers (mean age, 57.2 years) without a history of cancer. Because almost 25 percent of the baseline population had a history of CVD, the only outcomes considered in this report were cancer, all-cause mortality, and harms.[59] PHS-I was conducted among 22,071 healthy male physicians (mean age, 53 years) in the United States.[61] WHS was conducted among 39,876 healthy female health professionals age 45 years or older.[62] NSCPS was conducted among residents of the city of Nambour in southeast Queensland, Australia who took part in a skin cancer prevention study (56% female; mean age, 48.7 years), of which nearly 27 percent had a history of skin cancer (i.e., BCC or SCC).[64] SCPS randomized 1,805 individuals (31% female; mean age, 63 years) at high risk for NMSC (i.e., a previous history of BCC or SCC) and was designed to examine whether a beta-carotene supplement would decrease the time to first reoccurrence and the number of new skin cancer cases.[63] CARET aimed to prevent lung cancer among two separate high-risk groups (n=18,314), asbestos-exposed workers and heavy smokers.[60] The asbestos-exposed group included all men, while the heavy smokers included men and women (34.3% of entire study population was female).

We rated five of the six trials as good quality.[59-62,64] Among the good-quality studies, adherence was relatively high in four trials, with 70 to 93 percent of participants taking at least 80 percent of the assigned supplements. Even though three trials were discontinued early, two due to null findings (PHS-I and WHS)[61,62] and the other due to the increased risk of developing lung cancer and mortality among its participants (CARET),[60] they were rated good quality. SCPS was rated fair because it did not report randomization or blinding procedures.[63]

CVD

Two RCTs (n=61,947) examined incidence of nonfatal MI and nonfatal stroke as primary outcomes and found no statistically significant effect from beta-carotene supplementation (**Table 14**).[61,62] Although there were more CVD-related deaths in the beta-carotene intervention groups in four of the five trials, none of the between-group differences were statistically significant.[60-64] There were also no significant effects on the incidence of diabetes mellitus among participants taking beta-carotene in PHS-I (RR, 0.99 [95% CI, 0.86 to 1.14])[65] or the ATBC trial (RR, 0.99 [95% CI, 0.85 to 1.15]; data not shown).[66]

Cancer

Four RCTs (n=109,394) reported cancer incidence with mixed results, largely due to populations studied (**Table 15**).[59-62] Any cancer (except NMSC) was the primary outcome for two trials (PHS-I and WHS), while the incidence of lung cancer was the primary outcome for the other two trials (CARET and ATBC). PHS-I and WHS found no effect of beta-carotene on the incidence of any cancer, including lung cancer, in average-risk adults (**Figure 3**),[61,62] while CARET and the ATBC trial found statistically significant increased incidence of lung cancer with beta-carotene supplementation after 4 and 6.1 years followup, respectively.[59,60] Participants in the ATBC trial and CARET were at high risk for lung cancer at baseline, as study investigators specifically recruited current heavy smokers or asbestos-exposed workers. The risk of developing lung cancer was mitigated with longer followup and was no longer statistically significant in either CARET or the ATBC trial after 10 and 11 years, respectively.

Beta-carotene supplementation had no statistically significant effect on breast,[62,67] prostate,[59,67,68] pancreatic,[62,68,69] stomach,[59,62,68] gastric,[70] urothelial,[71] renal cell,[71] uterine,[62] ovarian,[62] cervical,[62] brain,[62,68] head/neck,[67] oral/pharyngeal,[72] esophageal,[72] laryngeal,[72] kidney,[73] lymphoma,[62,67,68] leukemia,[62,67,68] and melanoma cancer incidence rates (data not shown).[62,68] PHS-I found a statistically significant increased risk for thyroid (p=0.003) and bladder (p=0.04) cancer among those randomized to receive beta-carotene after 12.9 years of followup (data not shown).[68] The ATBC trial, CARET, and WHS found no statistically significant difference in bladder cancer (data not shown).[59,62,67] WHS found no difference in the incidence of thyroid cancer among women after 4.1 years (data not shown).[62] The ATBC trial found a late effect on the overall incidence of colorectal cancer only during the 6 years posttrial (RR, 1.44 [95% CI, 1.09 to 1.90]),[73] while no other trials found a statistically significant effect on this cancer.[62,67,68] The variation of these site-specific cancer results most likely reflects the post hoc nature of the testing, variation in baseline risk among populations recruited for different study aims, and lower power for relatively rare cancers due to small sample sizes.

Cancer mortality was reported in six RCTs (n=112,820) with mixed results.[59-64] Four trials found no statistically significant difference with beta-carotene supplementation in the number of cancer-related deaths.[61-64] As with incidence, however, there were more lung cancer deaths among those randomized to receive beta-carotene than those who were not, especially among the two trials of high-risk participants (ATBC and CARET).[59,60] These harmful results, along with consideration of the negative effects on lung cancer prevention identified in the ATBC trial, led to the early discontinuation of CARET. Even with further followup in CARET, those who had been taking the beta-carotene in combination with vitamin A supplement were at an increased risk of lung cancer mortality (RR, 1.20 [95% CI, 1.01 to 1.43]).[74] In the two high-risk subgroups of this trial, only smokers had an increased risk of dying from lung cancer at 6 years of followup (RR, 1.21 [95% CI, 1.00 to 1.47]), not the asbestos-exposed workers (RR, 1.16 [95% CI, 0.77 to 1.75]). PHS-I, WHS, and SCPS did not show any statistically significant effects with beta-carotene supplementation on lung cancer mortality, probably due to the participants' low risk at baseline.[61,62,75]

Beta-carotene supplementation had no statistically significant effects on prostate,[76] colorectal,[77] pancreatic,[69] urothelial,[71] renal cell,[71] oral/pharyngeal,[72] esophageal,[72] and laryngeal cancer deaths (data not shown).[72]

All-Cause Mortality

All-cause mortality was reported in six RCTs (n=112,820) (**Table 16**).[59-64] Four RCTs showed no significant effect on all-cause mortality among participants taking beta-carotene (**Figure 4**). The only statistically significant increases were among the two trials (ATBC and CARET) that specifically recruited participants at risk for lung cancer (i.e., heavy smokers and/or asbestos-exposed workers).[59,60]

Harms

Few details on adverse events were reported in six beta-carotene trials (n=112,820).[59-64] PHS-I reported no major side effects associated with the intervention during the 12 years of followup.[61] In NSCPS, 8 percent of participants withdrew from the study due to symptoms attributed to the study tablets or were unwilling to take the tablets (65 in the intervention group vs. 64 in the control group).[64] Four percent of participants in SCPS stopped taking the study capsules due to capsule-related symptoms (49 in the intervention group vs. 31 in the control group) within the first 2 years of the study.[63]

Yellowing of the skin was the most commonly reported adverse event (**Table 17**). There were no statistically significant differences in the number of minor gastrointestinal symptoms (e.g., belching) or other minor side effects (e.g., headaches) in PHS-I,[61] WHS,[62] and CARET.[60]

In a post hoc analysis, the ATBC trial also examined the effect of beta-carotene supplementation on the incidence of hospital-treated pneumonia in male smokers and found no overall effect (RR, 0.98 [95% CI, 0.85 to 1.11]).[78] Men who started smoking at an older age (>20 years) and were assigned to receive beta-carotene were at a higher risk for pneumonia than those who started smoking at a younger age (p=0.004).

Vitamin E

Summary of Results

Six fair- to good-quality trials of vitamin E supplementation, alone or in combination with another supplement, met our inclusion criteria (n=120,335).[52,59,79-82] This is the largest set of studies on any supplement included in this report. No beneficial effects were seen on CVD, cancer, or all-cause mortality (**Table 18**).

Study Details

We identified six RCTs evaluating vitamin E (n=120,335) (**Appendix E Tables 1** and **2**).[52,59,79-82] The trial by Graat and colleagues, described previously in the multivitamin section, included a separate vitamin E arm.[52] This study was a small, good-quality RCT that randomized 652 men and women older than age 60 years to a multivitamin or vitamin E (200 mg daily) in a 2x2 factorial design. The main outcome for this trial was acute respiratory infection. The other five trials were ATBC (described previously),[59] PHS-II (described previously),[80] the Selenium and Vitamin E Cancer Prevention Trial (SELECT),[82] WHS (described previously),[81] and the Antioxidant Supplementations in Atherosclerosis Prevention (ASAP) study.[79]

The RCTs were all double-blind, placebo-controlled trials. We rated them as good quality, except for ASAP, which we rated fair because it did not specify blinding, randomization, or outcome assessment methods. Two of the trials had 2x2 factorial designs, randomizing participants to vitamin E (200 mg daily[52] or 30 mg daily[59]), another study supplement (a multivitamin[52] or beta-carotene), both, or placebo.[59] WHS had a 2x2x2 factorial design with three active intervention groups: vitamin E (600 IU every other day), beta-carotene (50 mg every other day), and aspirin (50 mg every other day).[81] PHS-II had a 2x2x2x2 factorial design with four active intervention groups: vitamin E (400 IU), vitamin C (500 mg), a multivitamin, or beta-carotene.[83] SELECT randomized participants to selenium (200 mcg), vitamin E (400 IU), both, or placebo.[82] ASAP also had a 2x2 factorial design that randomized 520 individuals with hypercholesterolemia (51% female) to vitamin E (91 mg), vitamin C (50 mg), both, or placebo in order to prevent atherosclerosis.

Three trials included only men and one included only women. The ATBC trial was conducted in 29,133 male smokers (mean age, 57.2 years) to prevent lung cancer;[59] PHS-II was conducted in 14,641 male physicians (mean age, 64.3 years) to prevent CVD and cancer. SELECT was conducted in 35,533 men older than age 50 years to prevent prostate cancer.[82] Only one trial (WHS) was conducted in women: 39,876 female health professionals (mean age, 55 years) to prevent CVD and cancer.[81]

CVD

Three trials (n=90,050) reported cardiovascular incidence and mortality (**Figure 2**).[80-82] As reported in a secondary analysis, SELECT found no evidence of any impact on any "serious" cardiovascular event (including death) from vitamin E supplementation alone or combined with selenium (**Table 19**).[82] PHS-II and WHS reported incidence rates for nonfatal MI and nonfatal stroke (both primary outcomes in addition to CVD death) and showed no statistically significant effect.[80,81] In PHS-II, there was an excess number of hemorrhagic strokes observed among those assigned to vitamin E compared with those not assigned to vitamin E (39 vs. 23 events; p=0.036).[80] The other two studies (WHS and SELECT) found no statistically significant differences in the number of hemorrhagic strokes with vitamin E supplementation (data not shown).[81,82] This difference among these trials likely reflects the small number of these specific events and the post hoc analysis.

A subgroup analysis in WHS found that older women (age 65 years and older) who had received vitamin E supplementation had a significant reduction in major cardiovascular events (p=0.009), while younger women (ages 45 to 54 years and 55 to 64 years) had no effect.[81]

The same three trials also reported on CVD mortality (n=90,050) (**Table 19**).[80-82] The CVD mortality rate in WHS was lower in the intervention group (RR, 0.76 [95% CI, 0.59 to 0.98]), but the overall 10-year mortality rate was very low (0.6%).[81] The mortality rates for fatal MI and strokes did not reach statistical significance. The between-group differences in CVD mortality rates in the two all-male trials (PHS-II and SELECT) did not reach statistical significance.[80,82] The benefit seen in WHS could well reflect a chance finding given the small number of events, or the biological effects of vitamin E may be different in women than men. This speculation is supported by different effects of aspirin for primary CVD prevention in men and women.[84,85]

Cancer

Any and/or site-specific cancer incidence was reported as a primary outcome in four RCTs (n=119,183) (**Table 20**).[59,81-83] The ATBC study reported significantly less prostate cancer incidence among participants randomized to vitamin E than those who were not randomized to vitamin E at 6.1 and 8 years followup (p=0.002).[73,76] These differences did not persist at longer followup times (i.e., after 11 and 14 years),[73] although no information is known about supplement use after the trial ended. SELECT and PHS-II also reported prostate cancer incidence and neither found any evidence of an effect at the end of their trials.[82,83] In an extended followup of SELECT participants, however, there were significantly more prostate cancer cases in the vitamin E only group than in placebo (p=0.008).[82] SELECT and PHS-II each had more than twice the number of prostate cancer cases than did ATBC, which may explain the different results. Certainly the extended SELECT results call into question any conclusion that vitamin E might protect against prostate cancer.

None of the trials reported a statistically significant effect of vitamin E on the incidence of all cancers combined (**Figure 3**)[81-83] or of other site-specific cancers, including lung,[59,73,81-83] breast,[81] colorectal,[59,73,77,81-83] gastric,[70] stomach,[59,73,81] kidney,[73] pancreatic,[69,83] urothelial,[71] renal cell,[71] oral/pharyngeal,[72] esophageal,[72] laryngeal,[72] epithelial,[83] leukemia,[83] bladder,[59,83,86] lymphoma,[83] and melanoma (data not shown).[83]

Three RCTs (n=90,050) reported overall cancer mortality and none of the between-group differences were significant (**Table 20**).[81-83] Vitamin E supplementation showed no statistically significant effects on lung,[59,73,82,83] colorectal,[77,82,83] pancreatic,[69,83] bladder,[83] urothelial,[71] esophageal,[72] and laryngeal cancer[72] mortality rates or mortality rates from lymphoma,[83] leukemia,[83] and melanoma[83] (data not shown). In ATBC, there were significantly fewer male smokers dying from prostate cancer with vitamin E supplementation than those without vitamin E supplementation (RR, 0.59 [95% CI, 0.35 to 0.99]).[76] PHS-II, however, found no significant differences in prostate cancer mortality rates (RR, 1.01 [95% CI, 0.64 to 1.58])[83] and SELECT reported no prostate cancer deaths in any of the vitamin E arms (only one death in the control group).[82] Again, the number of prostate cancer deaths is small in all three trials, so chance may be playing a role. Also, in the ATBC trial, half of the men taking vitamin E were also taking beta-carotene and may have died from lung cancer before any prostate cancer became evident.

All-Cause Mortality

Five trials reported all-cause mortality data (n=119,703) (**Figure 4**).[59,79-82] The small ASAP study reported four deaths among those receiving vitamin E (either alone or combined with vitamin C) and one in the placebo group.[79] The other four trials found no difference in all-cause mortality between intervention and control groups (**Table 21**).[59,80-82]

Harms

All six vitamin E trials reported on harms (n=120,355).[52,59,79-82] PHS-II reported no differences between groups in observed adverse events, including bleeding, gastrointestinal symptoms, fatigue, drowsiness, skin discoloration, rashes, and migraines.[80] As discussed previously, there was a significantly greater risk of hemorrhagic stroke among participants receiving vitamin E supplementation in PHS-II (p=0.036), but this was not seen in the other two trials (WHS and SELECT). WHS reported a slight increase in epistaxis (RR, 1.06 [95% CI, 1.01 to 1.11]), but no other differences between groups in hematuria, gastrointestinal bleeding, or bruising.[81]

The study by Graat and colleagues evaluated the effect of vitamin E on respiratory tract infections in elderly men and women.[52] While supplementation had no significant effect on the incidence of infection (RR, 1.12 [95% CI, 0.88 to 1.25]), the severity of infection was worse among those who did not receive vitamin E, with longer duration, more symptoms, more fever, and more restricted activity. The ATBC trial also examined the effect of vitamin E supplementation on the incidence of hospital-treated pneumonia in male smokers and found no overall effect (RR, 1.00 [95% CI, 0.88 to 1.14]).[78] Men who started smoking at an older age (>20 years) and were assigned to receive vitamin E were at a lower risk for pneumonia than those who started smoking at a younger age (p=0.0007).[78] Among those who started smoking before age 21 years, those who weighed less than 60 kg or greater than 100 kg, had a greater dietary vitamin C intake (i.e., above the median), and had a lack of exercise were associated with a statistically significant increased risk for pneumonia.[87,88]

SELECT reported no statistically significant increase in alopecia, dermatitis, halitosis, nail changes, or fatigue among participants randomized to vitamin E alone or in combination with selenium when compared with placebo.[82] In the ASAP study, there was a similar number of dropouts due to severe and nonsevere adverse events between groups; no further details were provided.[79]

Selenium

Summary of Results

Two fair- to good-quality RCTs (n=36,845) examining selenium, either alone or in combination with another study supplement, found no effect on CVD or all-cause mortality.[82,89] The results were mixed for cancer prevention (**Table 22**). The Nutritional Prevention of Cancer Study (NPC) found a statistically significant decreased risk of cancer incidence and cancer-related mortality among participants randomized to selenium ($p<0.05$), with decreased risk of prostate and colorectal cancer specifically ($p<0.05$ for each).[89] The benefits decreased over time. SELECT, however, found no effect of selenium supplementation, either alone or in combination with vitamin E, on incidence of any site-specific cancer or all cancer combined, or on cancer mortality.[82] The differences in results between trials may be attributed to a number of factors, including the lower quality rating of NPC and the different inclusion criteria. In addition, NPC's participants were drawn from a geographical area known to have low soil selenium levels (eastern United States). In a post hoc analysis, the benefits were seen only in men in the lowest tertile of selenium levels at baseline, so any benefits may reflect treatment of selenium deficiency. No apparent harms from selenium supplementation were identified in three trials (n=37,346).

Study Details

Three trials (n=37,346) of selenium supplementation met our inclusion criteria: NPC,[89,90] SELECT, and the U.K. Prevention of Cancer by Intervention with Selenium (U.K. PRECISE) (**Appendix E Tables 1** and **2**).[82] The fair-quality NPC recruited 1,312 men (75%) and women (25%) with a history of at least two SCCs or BCCs of the skin who lived in areas of the United States known to have low levels of environmental selenium.[89] The mean age of participants was 63 years and 28 percent were current smokers. The main hypothesis of the study, that selenium supplementation at nutritional levels (200 mcg daily) would reduce the risk of BCC and SCC, was not supported by the results. Below we report secondary cancer and cardiovascular outcomes and safety data. We rated NPC as having fair quality due to its lack of blinding and randomization methods. As discussed previously, the good-quality SELECT randomized 35,533 men older than age 50 years to selenium (200 mcg/d), vitamin E (400 IU/d), both, or placebo to prevent prostate cancer.[82] The good-quality U.K. PRECISE pilot trial randomized 501 older adults (mean age, 67.5 years; 47.4% female) to 100, 200, or 300 mcg of selenium or placebo.[91] Only harms from selenium supplementation have been reported.

CVD

Neither SELECT nor NPC (as reported in secondary analyses) found any evidence of effects with selenium supplementation, either alone or in combination with vitamin E, on CVD (n=36,845) (**Table 23**, **Figure 2**).[82,89] NPC specifically examined the incidence of coronary heart disease (i.e., fatal and nonfatal MI, coronary bypass graft surgery, or percutaneous transluminal coronary angioplasty), cerebrovascular events (i.e., stroke or carotid endarterectomy), or CVD-related death among participants without a history of CVD (n=1,004), while SELECT collected self-reported "serious" cardiac events. There were no statistically significant differences in the incidence of diabetes mellitus between either of the selenium and placebo arms at either followup time points in SELECT (data not shown).[82]

Cancer

The two selenium trials had mixed cancer outcomes (n=36,845) (**Table 24, Figure 3**).[82,89] SELECT found no evidence of effects on the incidence of prostate, lung, colorectal, or any cancer overall at or beyond 5 years of followup with selenium supplementation.[82] In contrast, NPC reported significant 6-year decreases in any cancer,[89,92] prostate,[89,92,93] lung,[89,92] and colorectal cancer.[89,92] However, with longer-term followup through the end of the blinded trial (over 7 years), the differences in lung[90,94] and colorectal cancer[90] became statistically nonsignificant. The risk for any cancer[90] and prostate cancer[90,95] lessened but remained significant. The differences in results between trials may be attributed to a number of factors, including the lower quality rating for NPC and the different inclusion criteria (history of NMSC for NPC, normal prostate examination and prostate-specific antigen level in SELECT). Perhaps most importantly, NPC's participants were drawn from a geographical area known to have low soil selenium levels (eastern United States) and the benefits were seen only in men in the lowest tertile of baseline selenium, so if the apparent benefits are true, they may reflect treatment of selenium deficiency. NPC was a much smaller trial (n=1,312) than SELECT (n=35,533) and pooled analyses show no difference in cancer outcomes (RR for any cancer incidence, 0.91 [95% CI, 0.70 to 1.18]) (**Figure 3**).

NPC found no effect of selenium supplementation on cancers of the head/neck,[89,90,92] bladder,[89,90,92] esophagus,[89,90,92] or breast[89,90,92] or on melanoma[89,90] or leukemia/lymphoma at any followup times.[89,90] NPC also reported a significant decline in cancer mortality for the intervention group at 6 years[89,92] and 7.5 years followup.[90] Lung cancer deaths were also significantly less in the selenium group than the placebo group after 6 years.[89,92] SELECT found no effect of selenium supplementation on any or site-specific cancer mortality.[82]

All-Cause Mortality

There were no differences in mortality in either NPC or SELECT with selenium supplementation (n=36,485) (**Table 25, Figure 4**).[82,89]

Harms

NPC reported no dermatologic signs of selenium toxicity (n=1,312); however, 35 participants withdrew from the study due to adverse effects (e.g., gastrointestinal upset).[89] For selenium alone, SELECT found statistically significant increased risks of alopecia (RR, 1.28 [95% CI, 1.01 to 1.62]) and mild dermatitis (RR, 1.17 [95% CI, 1.00 to 1.35]).[82] When combined with vitamin E, there were no differences in the incidence of alopecia or mild dermatitis compared with placebo. The U.K. PRECISE trial found no serious harms; stomach or abdominal discomfort were the most frequently reported adverse events and they were equally distributed among arms.[91]

Vitamin A

Summary of Results

Three fair- to good-quality RCTs (n=20,958) and two cohort studies (n=107,040) examined the efficacy and/or safety of vitamin A supplementation, either alone or in combination with other study supplements (**Table 26**).[53,60,96-98] None of the studies reported CVD incidence. The only RCT (CARET) reporting cancer incidence found a statistically significant increased risk for lung cancer, but not all or other site-specific cancer, among those randomized to receive vitamin A with beta-carotene. This increased risk may be attributed to the beta-carotene supplement, as one other beta-carotene trial also showed statistically significant increased risk for lung cancer among participants at an increased risk at baseline for lung cancer (i.e., smokers) (both trials previously discussed). CARET also found an increased risk of death with the combination supplement, but the only other RCT reporting all-cause mortality with vitamin A supplementation did not (SKICAP-AK). Once again, this may be attributed to the participants' baseline risk. The other included trials found no statistically significant harms in the vitamin A groups. One cohort study among women found a statistically increased risk of harm among past vitamin A users, while the other cohort study did not.

Study Details

As discussed previously, we identified one good-quality RCT (CARET) that examined the efficacy of vitamin A supplementation (25,000 IU daily) in combination with beta-carotene (30 mg daily) to prevent cancer or CVD.[60] This study was conducted among 18,314 smokers and asbestos-exposed workers (mean age, 57.5 years). No other vitamin A efficacy trials were identified. We identified two fair-quality RCTs examining the safety of vitamin A supplementation, SKICAP-S/B[98] and SKICAP-AK.[97]

The SKICAP trials were both randomized, double-blind, placebo-controlled trials designed to evaluate the efficacy of vitamin A supplementation to prevent the incidence of NMSC. SKICAP-S/B (n=347) focused on a population at high risk for recurrence of NMSC by requiring a history of four or more pathologically confirmed BCCs or SCCs for inclusion.[98] Participants were randomized to receive either 25,000 IU of vitamin A or a placebo once a day for 3 years and were evaluated every 6 months by study staff. A third arm was also included for isotretinion (a vitamin A derivative) (5 to 10 mg). We did not report those outcomes, as isotretinion is not considered a dietary supplement and is used primarily to treat acne. SKICAP-AK (n=2,297) was similar in design to SKICAP-S/B, but focused on a population at moderate risk for developing a recurrence of NMSC.[97] Participants were required to have a history of 10 or more pathologically confirmed actinic keratoses (most recent diagnosis within the preceding year) and a pathologically confirmed record of at most one prior SCC or BCC. While both of these trials report skin cancer outcomes, we did not consider those results because neither trial would be considered primary prevention by design; we considered only their all-cause mortality and harms data. We rated both the SKICAP trials as having fair quality due to the lack of randomization methods and allocation concealment.

Two good-quality prospective cohort studies were included for harms: the Iowa Women's Health Study (IWHS)[96] and NHS.[53] Details of these studies are reported in **Appendix E Tables 1** and **2**.

IWHS (n=34,703) and NHS (n=72,337) were both good-quality large prospective cohorts of postmenopausal women aiming to assess the effectiveness of vitamin supplements in preventing hip fractures.[53,96] In addition to hip fractures, IWHS evaluated the impact of vitamin supplements on cancer, diabetes, and hypertension. We only considered those results related to harms, however, due to study design.

CVD

As mentioned previously, CARET did not evaluate CVD incidence, and there were no significant differences between groups in the number of CVD-related deaths after 4 years of supplementation and during the 6-year postintervention followup (n=18,314) (**Table 14**).

Cancer

As mentioned previously, there were more incident lung cancer cases and deaths in the combination supplement group than in the placebo group in CARET (n=18,314) after 4 years of followup (p=0.02) (**Table 15**). With further followup (6 years postintervention), the risk of developing lung cancer was no longer significant (p=0.13), but the related mortality risk was not mitigated. There were no statistically significant differences in the incidence and mortality rates of other site-specific cancers (e.g., prostate, breast, and colorectal).

All-Cause Mortality

Two RCTs reported all-cause mortality (n=20,611) (**Figure 4**). The number of deaths in SKICAP-AK was similar between treatment arms.[97] After 5 years of followup, 5.4 percent of the intervention group and 4.5 percent of the control group had died, with a mortality ratio of 1.08 (95% CI, 0.78 to 1.50). In contrast, CARET reported more deaths in the combination supplement group than the placebo group (RR, 1.17 [95% CI, 1.03 to 1.33]) after 4 years, but with longer followup, the difference was no longer significant (p=0.07 after 6 years postintervention) (**Table 16**). These trials differed in many ways (e.g., size, baseline risk of lung cancer), so this difference in all-cause mortality may simply reflect the clinical heterogeneity between trials, which included the use of beta-carotene supplementation in CARET.

Harms

All five included vitamin A studies reported harms (n=127,998).[53,60,96-98] Two cohort studies examined associations between hip fractures and vitamin A intake, since high vitamin A intake contributes to osteoporosis by decreasing bone mass.[99,100] NHS reported an increase in hip fractures among those who used vitamin A supplements currently (RR, 1.40 [95% CI, 0.99 to 1.99]) or in the past (RR, 1.34 [95% CI, 1.01 to 1.76]) compared with those not taking vitamin A.[53] The risk of hip fracture was also increased in a subgroup of women using vitamin A supplements but with low dietary intake of the vitamin (RR, 1.75 [95% CI, 1.09 to 2.80]). This study also found that dietary vitamin A intake increased hip fracture risk.

Similarly, IWHS found an increase in hip fractures that did not quite achieve statistical significance (RR, 1.18 [95% CI, 0.99 to 1.41]) in those taking supplements containing vitamin A.[96] During a mean length of followup of 9.5 person-years, there were 6,502 fractures, including

525 hip fractures. Unlike NHS, this study also reported the association of vitamin A supplements with risk of any fracture and found no relationship (RR, 1.00 [95% CI, 0.95 to 1.05]). In both of these studies, investigators relied on self-reported information via questionnaires and were unable to confirm the incidence of a fracture or the site of fracture. Ingesting toxic amounts of vitamin A has adverse skeletal effects in humans and animals, so the results of these two observational studies raise a concern.[53]

In two trials reporting harms of vitamin A supplements (SKICAP-AK and SKICAP-S/B), no serious adverse events were reported.[97,98] In SKICAP-AK, harmful symptoms were rarely reported and were similar in frequency between both study groups through 5 years of followup.[97] Symptoms that led to cessation of the medication were also not significantly different between groups. The SKICAP-S/B trial analyzed adverse events by focusing on the number of patients experiencing clinical toxicity (level 2 or greater).[98] Similar to SKICAP-AK, occurrences of participants experiencing clinical toxicity were rare, and though instances of toxicity were slightly more common in participants taking vitamin A, the difference was reported to not be significant. CARET also reported no differences in the incidence of adverse effects (e.g., headaches) between those taking the combination supplement and placebo, and only 0.3 percent reported yellowing of skin of grade 3 or higher (**Table 17**).[60] There was also no evidence of systemic toxicity from vitamin A supplementation.

Vitamin C

Summary of Results

Two good- to fair-quality RCTs (n=15,161) examining vitamin C, either alone or in combination with another study supplement, found no effect on preventing CVD, cancer, or all-cause mortality (**Table 27**).[79,80] There were also no differences in harms.

Study Details

We identified one good-quality RCT examining the efficacy of vitamin C in preventing CVD and cancer (PHS-II),[80] along with one fair-quality RCT (ASAP) examining the safety of vitamin C supplementation (n=15,161) (**Appendix E Tables 1** and **2**).[79] Both studies have been previously described. PHS-II evaluated the cancer and cardiovascular outcomes for male physicians (age 55 years and older) taking vitamin C (500 mg once a day) against those not taking vitamin C (part of a 2x2x2x2 factorial design).[80] ASAP was a double-blind, 2x2 factorial-designed trial focusing on patients with hypercholesterolemia (serum cholesterol of ≥5.0 mmol/L) ages 45 to 69 years.[79] The vitamin C arms of the trial included participants taking slow-release vitamin C (250 mg twice a day), either alone (n=130) or in combination with vitamin E (n=130) (91 mg twice a day), over 3 years compared with placebo (n=130).

CVD

One good-quality study (PHS-II) (n=14,641) evaluated the impact of vitamin C supplementation on the primary prevention of major cardiovascular events (nonfatal stroke, nonfatal MI, and CVD death).[80] Over an average followup of 8 years, there was no significant difference in the incidence of any major cardiovascular event between those taking vitamin C and those not taking the vitamin (HR, 0.99 [95% CI, 0.89 to 1.11]) (**Table 28**, **Figure 2**). Specifically, there were no significant differences in the incidence of MI (p=0.65) or stroke (p=0.21). Death from any CVD event was similar between groups (p=0.86).

Cancer

PHS-II also evaluated the impact of vitamin C supplementation on the primary prevention of cancer (n=14,641) (**Table 29**, **Figure 3**).[83] There was no significant difference in any or site-specific cancer incidence between those taking vitamin C and those not taking the supplement (HR, 1.01 [95% CI, 0.92 to 1.10]). The incidence and mortality rates of lung, prostate, and colorectal cancer did not differ significantly between the two groups. The number of other cancer (e.g., bladder, epithelial, pancreatic, lymphoma, leukemia, and melanoma) cases and deaths reported were similar between the two groups as well. Death from any type of cancer was similar between groups (p=0.53).

All-Cause Mortality

Both PHS-II and the ASAP trial (n=15,161) reported all-cause mortality data and found no effect (**Table 30**, **Figure 4**). The ASAP trial (n=520) reported one death in each vitamin C arm (alone or in combination with vitamin E) over a 3-year study period.[79] The deaths in the intervention group were from subarachnoid hemorrhage or complications of carotid endartectomy, while the single death in the control group was from cardiac dysrhythmia. During PHS-II's 8-year study period (n=14,641), there were 857 deaths in the vitamin C group and 804 deaths in those not taking the vitamin (HR, 1.07 [95% CI, 0.97 to 1.18]).

Harms

None of the studies identified reported on adverse events from vitamin C supplementation. In ASAP, there were a similar number of dropouts due to severe and nonsevere adverse events between groups; no further details were provided.[79]

Folic Acid

Summary of Results

One fair-quality RCT (n=1,021) examining folic acid for preventing colorectal adenoma found no effect on MI, strokes, or all-cause mortality, but significantly more noncolorectal cancers in the intervention group than the placebo group (p=0.02) (**Table 31**).[101] The excess in noncolorectal cancer cases was attributed to the higher number of prostate cancers in the intervention group than the placebo group (p=0.02).

Study Details

Only one study of folic acid supplementation met the inclusion criteria: the Aspirin/Folate Polyp Prevention Study (AFPPS).[101,102] This double-blind, placebo-controlled RCT recruited 1,021 adults ages 21 to 80 years with a history of colorectal adenoma and randomized them to folic acid (1 mg daily) or placebo, then separately randomized them to receive aspirin (81 or 325 mg daily) or placebo (3x2 factorial design) (**Appendix E Tables 1** and **2**). The study was of fair quality because the relevant outcomes were based on secondary analyses. The main trial found no evidence that folic acid reduced colorectal adenoma incidence and there was some evidence of increased higher-grade adenoma or invasive colorectal cancer; however, these results are not considered in this report, as the study population included individuals with a previous colorectal adenoma. The study is included here for CVD, noncolorectal cancer, and prostate cancer outcomes only.

CVD

AFPPS (n=1,021) reported few MIs and strokes, both categorized as adverse events (i.e., a secondary outcome), 10.8 years after randomization; incident rates did not differ between the intervention and control groups (p>0.25 for each outcome).[101]

Cancer

In AFPPS (n=1,021), there were significantly more noncolorectal cancer cases in the intervention group than the control group (p=0.02) (**Figure 3**).[101] In a secondary analysis, AFPPS reported prostate cancer incidence among the 643 men included in the study who were randomized to receive folic acid or placebo (i.e., men randomly assigned to aspirin only were not analyzed).[102] Thirty-four prostate cancers were diagnosed; the adjusted probability of this diagnosis was 9.7 percent in the intervention group and 3.3 percent in the control group (HR, 2.58 [95% CI, 1.14 to 5.86]) after 10.8 years. The study investigators attributed the higher rate of noncolorectal cancers in the intervention group to the excess of prostate cancer cases.[101]

All-Cause Mortality

AFPPS (n=1,021) reported all-cause mortality; 10 deaths occurred in the intervention group and 19 in the control group (p=0.09) (**Figure 4**).[101]

Harms

Except for the increased risk of prostate cancer noted previously, AFPPS (n=1,021) did not report on additional harms with folic acid supplementation.[101]

Vitamin D

Summary of Results

The beneficial and harmful effects of vitamin D on CVD and cancer were studied in three fair- to good-quality trials (n=8,106) (**Table 32**).[103-105] None of the trials reported on CVD incidence; the only trial that reported on CVD mortality found no effect of vitamin D supplementation. The same trial also found no effect on cancer incidence, cancer mortality, or all-cause mortality. Vitamin D was associated with few adverse effects.

Study Details

We identified two RCTs examining the effects of vitamin D (n=7,978) on cancer, CVD, and/or all-cause mortality: the Randomized Evaluation of Calcium or Vitamin D (RECORD)[103] and a UK-based study by Trivedi and colleagues (**Appendix E Tables 1** and **2**).[104] The RECORD trial, a 2x2 factorial study, examined the effects of vitamin D_3 (800 IU daily) and calcium (1,000 mg daily) supplementation.[103] It randomized 5,292 participants (mean age, 75 years) with a history of a fragility fracture; 85 percent were female. The study by Trivedi and colleagues examined the effects of 100,000 units of vitamin D_3 administered orally every 4 months for 5 years.[104] It randomized 2,686 healthy participants (mean age, 75 years; 24% women) living in the community; about three quarters were physicians from the British Doctors Study.[104] Both trials were also designed to examine fracture outcomes. A third study, by Dean and colleagues, was a short, small trial testing the effects of vitamin D 5,000 IU daily on cognitive and emotional function in young adults.[105] We included its data on harms. This trial included 128 healthy men and women recruited at the University of Queensland with a mean age of 22 years.

CVD

Two trials (n=7,979) of vitamin D supplementation reported on CVD incidence (**Table 33**).[104,106] The RECORD trial (n=5,292) included fatal CVD as a primary outcome. This trial found no statistically significant effect on any cardiovascular events, MI, stroke, or fatal event between participants receiving vitamin D and those who were not.[103] It did, however, find a statistically significant decreased risk for cardiac failure among those taking vitamin D.[106] Trivedi and colleagues (n=2,686) also reported CVD incidence (a primary outcome) and related deaths and found no effect with vitamin D supplementation.[104]

Cancer

Two trials reported on cancer incidence as primary outcomes (n=7,978). The RECORD trial found similar rates of any and site-specific cancer between those randomized to receive vitamin D and those who were not (**Table 34**, **Figure 3**); there were also no statistically significant effects on cancer-related deaths.[103] Trivedi and colleagues (n=2,686) also found no effect on cancer incidence or cancer-related deaths with vitamin D supplementation, except on colon cancer-related deaths in women (p=0.04) but not men (p=0.96).[104]

All-Cause Mortality

Two trials provided all-cause mortality data (n=7,978) (**Figure 4**).[103,104] There were fewer deaths in the vitamin D arm of the Trivedi study than in the placebo arm; however, the age-adjusted RR was not statistically significant (**Table 35**).[104] In RECORD, similar mortality rates were seen among those randomized to vitamin D and those randomized to no vitamin D (31.6% vs. 33.3%).[103] The overall test for a main effect of vitamin D on all-cause mortality was not significant (HR, 0.93 [95% CI, 0.85 to 1.02]).

Harms

Vitamin D supplementation was not associated with any statistically significant harms among two trials (n=5,420).[103,105] One control participant in the study by Dean and colleagues reported one episode of transient rectal bleeding, and there were no significant differences between groups on the Treatment Emergent Symptom Scale, a 31-item self-report questionnaire capturing a range of potential adverse effects, after 6 weeks of followup (p=0.26).[105] In the RECORD trial, renal insufficiency developed in seven participants, renal stones in four, and hypercalcemia in 21 (data were not stratified by arm), but there were no significant differences between the treatment arms after 5 years followup.[103] There were no significant differences in serious adverse events between groups, with 13.7 percent of those randomized to receive vitamin D and 14.5 percent of those randomized to receive no vitamin D reporting side effects.[107]

Vitamin D and Calcium

Summary of Results

We identified one fair-quality and one good-quality trial examining the combination supplement of vitamin D and calcium (n=37,462) (**Table 36**).[108,109] The simplest interpretation of the results from these two trials is that the combination supplement most likely has no effect on CVD or cancer. The best evidence of a benefit from vitamin D comes from the study by Lappe and colleagues, conducted in rural Nebraska, where vitamin D levels are known to be low, and used a dose of vitamin D that was 2.5 times greater than that used in WHI; this study found a statistically significant decreased risk of any cancer with supplement use (p=0.018). This was a small study (n=1,180), however, and we rated it as only fair quality.

Study Details

We identified one good-quality[108] and one fair-quality[109] RCT that studied the combination of vitamin D and calcium (**Appendix E Tables 1** and **2**). These trials were designed to test the effects of this supplementation on fracture risk and mortality; CVD was a prespecified outcome for WHI.[108] The study by Lappe and colleagues recruited 1,180 women (mean age, 62 years) from rural Nebraska, where vitamin D levels are known to be low but not necessarily deficient.[109] It randomized women to receive calcium alone (1,400 to 1,500 mg daily), vitamin D (1,000 IU or 25 mcg daily) in combination with calcium, or placebo. We rated this trial as fair quality because the reports lacked detail about allocation concealment, blinding of outcome ascertainment, and differential followup. WHI was also limited to women (mean age, 68 years) but was much larger, with 36,282 participants randomized to vitamin D (200 IU or 5 mcg twice daily) and calcium (500 mg twice daily) or placebo. We rated it as good quality.[108] It was designed to primarily examine vitamin D and calcium supplementation for preventing hip fractures and secondarily other fractures and colorectal cancer.

CVD

Only WHI (n=26,282) reported CVD incidence and mortality (primary outcomes included MI, angina, stroke, and cardiovascular-related death) and found no effect with the combination supplement (**Table 37; Figure 2**).[108] The WHI investigators also examined the incidence of diabetes and found no effect with supplementation (HR, 1.01 [95% CI, 0.94 to 1.10]; data not shown).[110]

Cancer

Two trials (n=37,462) reported on cancer incidence and mortality with mixed results (**Table 38**; **Figure 3**).[108,109] The study by Lappe and colleagues found a statistically significant reduction in the incidence of any cancer (p=0.013) after 4 years of vitamin D in combination with calcium supplementation.[109] This result is similar in magnitude to the findings in the calcium-only arm (discussed below), but for calcium the difference was not statistically significant. There were fewer breast, colon, lung, uterine, lymph, leukemia, and myeloma cancer cases in the intervention group than the placebo group (data not shown). WHI found no effect of the combination supplement on any cancer incidence (total or site-specific) or mortality rates.[108] A post hoc subgroup analysis of the WHI data showed that vitamin D in combination with calcium supplementation was associated with lower total cancer and breast cancer incidence among women who were not taking either supplement at baseline.[111]

All-Cause Mortality

Only WHI (n=36,282) reported on all-cause mortality. It found no effect with the combination supplement after 7 years of followup (**Table 39**, **Figure 4**).

Harms

Two trials reported on harms (n=37,462). The Lappe study reported no serious supplement-related adverse events and found no differences between groups for any outcome, including renal calculi, which was the most serious adverse event reported.[109] WHI reported a small increase in kidney stones in the combination supplement group compared with the placebo group (449 vs. 381; HR, 1.17 [95% CI, 1.02 to 1.34]); no other statistically significant different adverse outcomes were reported.[108] WHI also reported no statistically significant difference in the number of hip or total fractures (data not shown).[112]

Calcium

Summary of Results

Four trials (n=8,873) of calcium found no effect on overall CVD, cancer, or all-cause mortality (**Table 40**).[103,113,114] When data from two studies were pooled, calcium supplementation was associated with an increased risk of developing colorectal cancer (unadjusted Peto OR, 1.71 [95% CI, 1.08 to 2.72]) (**Appendix G**, **Figure 7**). Calcium supplementation was also frequently associated with side effects (e.g., constipation). Only one trial reported a significant increase in hip fractures in the calcium group, but it also reported fewer fractures at other sites, so the overall fracture rates were similar between treatment groups. None of the other RCTs reported differences between groups on fracture rates.[115]

Study Details

We identified four fair-quality RCTs that reported data on CVD, cancer, or both after calcium supplementation (**Appendix E Tables 1** and **2**): the Auckland Calcium Study (ACS),[113] the Calcium Polyp Prevention Study (CPPS),[114] the RECORD trial (discussed previously),[103] and the study conducted in Nebraska by Lappe and colleagues (discussed previously).[109]

The data we included from ACS and RECORD were secondary analyses of RCTs that were designed to evaluate fracture prevention.[103,113] The data we included from CPPS (cancer, strokes, and mortality) were secondary outcomes of an RCT designed to evaluate the impact of calcium supplementation on recurrent colorectal polyps.[114] The study by Lappe and colleagues primarily evaluated fracture prevention but also evaluated cancer incidence as a secondary endpoint. Its interventions included a combination supplementation (calcium in combination with vitamin D) and calcium alone.[109]

The 2x2 factorial-designed RECORD trial randomized participants age 70 years or older (n=5,292) to calcium (1,000 mg daily) or vitamin D_3 (800 IU daily) and comprised 85 percent women.[103] ACS recruited only postmenopausal women older than age 55 years (n=1,471) and randomized them to 1 g of daily calcium or placebo.[113] CPPS was designed to study the effects of calcium carbonate (1,200 mg daily) on colorectal adenoma recurrence (n=930); a secondary analysis investigated the risk of prostate cancer among the 672 men in the original trial.[114] The trial by Lappe and colleagues was conducted among 1,108 women (mean age, 67 years) in rural Nebraska, where vitamin D levels are generally low, and used a calcium dose of 1,500 mg daily.[109]

CVD

Two trials reported CVD incidence (n=2,110) (**Table 41**).[113,116] ACS measured any adverse cardiovascular event over 5 years and found more cases of adjudicated and verified MI and stroke in the calcium group, but the differences were not statistically significant. The composite endpoint of MI, stroke, and sudden death occurred in 60 women in the calcium group and 50 in the control group (p=0.32).[113] There was also no difference between groups on the incidence of other cardiovascular events (angina, other chest pain, or transient ischemic attack), which were reported only by participants or their families (data not shown). The CVD mortality rate was 50 percent lower in the calcium group, but there were only nine events and the difference was not significant.[113] In CPPS, there were no significant differences between groups in the number of participants hospitalized for stroke or cardiac disease (secondary endpoints).[116] The RECORD trial (n=5,292) included all "vascular" deaths, from cardiovascular, cerebrovascular, and other vascular disease. The RECORD investigators found a nonsignificant increase in vascular disease mortality (HR, 1.07 [95% CI, 0.92 to 1.24]) associated with calcium supplementation.

Cancer

Cancer outcomes were available from three trials (n=7,693) (**Table 42**).[103,109,114] The trial conducted by Lappe and colleagues reported a lower incidence of any cancer in the calcium group compared with the placebo group (3.8% vs. 6.9%); however, this finding was based on a total of 37 events and the difference did not attain statistical significance (p=0.063). The magnitude of the reduction was similar in the calcium plus D arm (reported previously), where the difference was significant. Site-specific cancer incidence rates were based on even fewer events and showed no statistically significant differences.[109] In RECORD, the rate of any cancer in participants randomized to receive calcium was similar to the rate in those who did not receive calcium; the number of site-specific cancers, however, was sometimes higher in the calcium group, but no statistical testing was performed. When data from two trials were pooled, calcium supplementation was associated with an increased risk for developing colorectal cancer (unadjusted Peto OR, 1.71 [95% CI, 1.08 to 2.72]) (**Appendix G**, **Figure 7**). This finding, however, is based on a total of only 73 cases (46 in intervention group and 27 in control group). CPPS found no significant difference between groups on any cancer incidence after 4 years. This trial also reported on prostate cancer incidence among the 672 men in the original trial and found no significant difference between the calcium and placebo groups after 10 years of followup.[114] The number of subjects hospitalized due to cancer was not significantly different between groups (data not shown).[116] Cancer mortality was reported only in RECORD (n=5,292) (**Table 38**); the main effect analysis of calcium supplementation showed no effect on any or site-specific cancer deaths.[103]

All-Cause Mortality

Three trials (n=7,693) found no statistically significant differences between groups for all-cause mortality (**Table 43**, **Figure 4**).[103,113,116]

Harms

Few adverse effects were reported by four trials (n=8,873).[103,109,113,114] The Lappe study reported no serious supplement-related adverse events and no differences between groups for any outcomes, including renal calculi, which was the most serious adverse event reported.[109] ACS found higher rates of constipation in the calcium group (18% vs. 11%; p=0.0002). The discontinuation rate was also higher (46% vs. 40%; p=0.02) and was attributed to the higher rates of constipation in the intervention group.[115] In CPPS, the frequency of digestive symptoms (e.g., constipation) did not differ between the calcium and placebo groups; three patients experienced urinary stones.[116] In addition, 3 percent of participants discontinued due to perceived toxicity during the study.

In RECORD, after 5 years of followup, study investigators noted poorer compliance with calcium supplementation that reflected more frequent decisions to stop supplementation due to gastrointestinal symptoms. More side effects were reported among participants taking calcium than those who were not (16.4% vs. 11.9%).[107] Renal insufficiency developed in seven participants, renal stones in four, and hypercalcemia in 21; these data were not reported separately by arm, but the investigators stated that there were no significant differences between the treatment arms after 5 years followup.

ACS also reported a significant increase in hip fractures in the calcium group: 17 in the calcium group and five in the control group (HR, 3.55 [95% CI, 1.31 to 9.63]). Fewer fractures occurred at other sites in the intervention group and the overall fracture rates were similar between the two groups (HR, 0.91 [95% CI, 0.71 to 1.17]).[115]

Summary of Pooled Data

Figures 2–4 summarize the results of this review across all supplements studied for any CVD incidence, any cancer incidence, and all-cause mortality. These figures make two main points. First, the opportunity for pooling is limited due to the limited number of studies. Second, there is little evidence of a dramatic effect of any of the supplements on any of the outcomes, even the one exception of any cancer incidence being lower in the two multivitamin supplement studies[49,50] (these figures depict both sexes, but the results for men only are nearly identical; data not shown). Additional figures are provided in **Appendix G**. The results from our meta-analysis may differ from those reported in original trials, as we used raw data and calculated unadjusted RRs and ORs.

Chapter 4. Discussion

Summary of Evidence

We conducted this systematic review to assist the USPSTF in updating its 2003 recommendation on using vitamin supplements to prevent CVD and cancer.[1] Our review included 26 studies (24 RCTs and two cohort studies) examining the benefits and harms of vitamins and minerals as primary prevention of CVD, cancer, and all-cause mortality (**Table 44**). For most of the supplements analyzed in this report, we found no evidence of an effect for nutritional doses on CVD, cancer, or all-cause mortality in healthy individuals with a presumed generally adequate diet based on study inclusion criteria and baseline serum levels. Other systematic reviews generally support this perspective.[117-127] For most supplements, however, there were a limited number of studies on which to base this conclusion, with the exception of vitamin E, which included six fair- to good-quality trials that all produced clearly null effects on these endpoints, consistent with the conclusions of other systematic reviews and meta-analyses.[128-132]

Another exception to this general conclusion are the two multivitamin studies, SU.VI.MAX and PHS-II (n=27,658), which found lower cancer incidence in men. Women were included only in SU.VI.MAX, which found a subgroup-specific benefit in men but not women (the interaction term was significant). When the data for men in these two studies were pooled, there was a statistically significant protective effect with multivitamin supplementation (unadjusted RR, 0.93 [95% CI, 0.87 to 0.99]; k=2; I^2=0.0%). From this ratio, we calculate that one cancer case would be prevented if 98 men used a daily multivitamin for 11.2 years (in PHS-II, NNT=83) to 12.5 years (in SU.VI.MAX, NNT=131).

SU.VI.MAX was a good-quality trial with randomization stratified by sex, which strengthens the validity of the comparison by sex. PHS-II was also rated good quality, with a large sample size and long followup. The small size of the effect in PHS-II and the lack of an effect in women in SU.VI.MAX suggest caution in overgeneralizing these results. Additional studies are warranted given the widespread use of multivitamin supplements in the United States, but the need to recruit many participants and follow them for a decade or more creates a large barrier to such research.

The authors of SU.VI.MAX speculate that the observed sex difference in multivitamin effects on cancer incidence may have been due to lower baseline antioxidant status in men than women. A baseline difference, however, was found only for beta-carotene—baseline levels of vitamins E and C, selenium, and zinc were similar in men and women.[49] Other behavioral or biological differences could modify the effects of antioxidant supplements on men and women, but with only one study showing the difference, speculation may be premature. Also, general scientific knowledge about sex-based biological differences is limited at best, since most basic cellular and molecular studies fail to consider or even identify the sex of the organism from which the study materials were derived.

While we provide pooled results for the multivitamin studies, direct comparison is made difficult by the design differences. PHS-II included a 32-component supplement, whereas the

SU.VI.MAX supplement contained only five components. The mean age in PHS-II was 64 years and in SU.VI.MAX was 49 years. Men in PHS-II took the multivitamin for over 11 years on average, whereas active treatment in SU.VI.MAX ended at 7.5 years. At 7.5 years, the benefit on cancer incidence in SU.VI.MAX was larger (RR, 0.69) than in PHS-II (RR, 0.92), but the latter was at 11.2 years. The RR for men in SU.VI.MAX at 12.5 years was closer to that in PHS-II (0.91), but the proportion of men who continued assigned treatment is unknown. The possibly larger effect in SU.VI.MAX could be attributed to the younger age, but PHS-II found trends favoring older individuals (>70 years) for both cancer incidence and CVD.[50,57]

Other evidence for sex differences in the results presented in this review is limited. Many of the studies included only one sex and the results were rarely stratified by sex among studies with mixed populations. One study of vitamin D supplementation showed a statistically significant protective effect against colon cancer death in women (p=0.04) but not men (p=0.96).[104] This analysis, however, was based on four deaths in the placebo group and none in the vitamin D group, so it is quite likely to be spurious (the sex interaction was not subjected to a formal test). When comparisons were made for other outcomes, no other sex differences were found.

One observational study, IWHS, addressed the question of multivitamin effects in postmenopausal women. IWHS was a good-quality longitudinal cohort study that began in 1986 and enrolled nearly 39,000 women.[133] While we excluded mortality data from all observational studies in the main review, this cohort study provides worthwhile context. In 2011, IWHS investigators compared the use of any one of 15 supplements in the 15,594 women who died during followup with those who were alive. The IWHS investigators found a small but significant increase in mortality among the multivitamin users. While IWHS reports findings by individual supplement, the participants were in fact taking a variable mix of supplements, complicating interpretation.

One more exception to lack of effects in supplement users is the potential harms of daily beta-carotene supplementation (range, 30 to 50 mg) among individuals at high risk for lung cancer. Two included trials (ATBC and CARET) examining the effect of beta-carotene supplementation (either alone or in combination with another supplement) specifically recruited and enrolled current heavy smokers,[59,60] asbestos-exposed workers, or both.[60] These two trials found a statistically significant increased risk for lung cancer and lung cancer death at various followup times, which led one of these studies to stop early.[60] Other beta-carotene studies stratified lung cancer incidence by smoking status after concerns were raised by the results from the ATBC trial and CARET. PHS-I found no statistically significant risk for developing lung cancer among current smokers (smoking level not reported) with beta-carotene supplementation (RR, 0.90 [95% CI, 0.58 to 1.40]).[61] WHS was unable to conduct any meaningful analyses of site-specific cancers among current smokers (smoking level not reported) due to the small number of participants who reported smoking at baseline (13%). WHS, however, did not find a statistically increased risk of invasive cancer among those assigned to receive beta-carotene.[62] While the difference in baseline lung cancer risk is the most likely explanation for the different outcomes in these studies, the dosage of the beta-carotene supplementation also differed. In the two trials in high-risk populations (ATBC and CARET), participants received 30 to 50 mg of beta-carotene daily, while in PHS-I and WHS, participants received 50 mg of beta-carotene every other day.

We identified a meta-analysis examining smoking status and the effect of beta-carotene on the incidence of lung cancer using pooled data from ATBC, CARET, PHS-I, and WHS.[134] Among current smokers, beta-carotene supplementation was significantly associated with an increased risk of lung cancer (OR, 1.24 [95% CI, 1.10 to 1.39]; k=4), but there was no effect on former smokers. A recent Cochrane review also found that individuals taking beta-carotene with a risk for lung cancer had a statistically significant increased risk of lung cancer incidence (RR, 1.11 [95% CI, 1.01 to 1.21]; k=4), lung cancer mortality (RR, 1.18 [95% CI, 1.01 to 1.38]; k=2), and all-cause mortality (RR, 1.09 [95% CI, 1.05 to 1.13]; k=2); no effect was seen among those not at risk for lung cancer.[135] No trend toward increased lung cancer incidence among individuals at high risk for lung cancer was seen in trials of supplements other than beta-carotene; there were also no significant effects on CVD, cancer, or mortality rates among those at high risk for lung cancer.

The effects of vitamin D and calcium, alone or in combination, on CVD and cancer were studied in five trials. Three trials provided data on calcium alone, but the results were mixed. RECORD and ACS showed some increase in CVD incidence, but ACS also showed a decrease in CVD mortality with calcium; none of the differences were significant. Cancer rates with calcium were lower in the Lappe study but higher in RECORD, and again neither difference was significant. Vitamin D plus calcium was specifically studied in two trials and the results were also mixed. Only one examined CVD incidence and found no effect. Both reported cancer outcomes and one smaller trial found a significant decrease in overall cancer incidence over 4 years, but the larger trial did not. Another trial (RECORD) examined vitamin D and calcium supplementation under a 2x2 factorial design and also found no effects with either supplementation. To further evaluate the independent effects of calcium on cancer, we reanalyzed the RECORD data comparing the calcium only arm to the placebo only arm (**Appendix F Tables 4–6; Appendix F Figures 1** and **2**). The point-estimate RRs were similar in the two analyses except, as expected, the CIs were wider in the calcium versus placebo comparison due to there being about half the number of events.

The simplest overall interpretation of the vitamin D and calcium results is that there is likely no effect on CVD or cancer. Wang and colleagues, in another systematic review of this topic, came to the same conclusion.[120] The data suggest, however, that the effects of calcium on these endpoints may be different than the effects of vitamin D. **Figure 4** shows the pooled analyses for all-cause mortality. There are only two vitamin D studies to pool, but together they show a trend toward lower mortality in the supplement groups (unadjusted RR, 0.94 [95% CI, 0.88 to 1.01]). In contrast, the point estimates for calcium are all greater than 1, though with large CIs. The lack of statistical significance makes this comparison speculative, but it does support the wisdom of conducting separate studies of calcium and vitamin D for the endpoints examined here.

In addition, several observers have recently raised the possibility of a harmful effect of calcium intake or supplementation on CVD outcomes. The ACS investigators have published two meta-analyses on calcium and CVD, in 2010[136] and 2011.[137] The 2011 meta-analysis includes some of the studies in the 2010 meta-analysis, plus a reanalysis of the WHI vitamin D and calcium study.[111] These analyses concluded that calcium supplementation is associated with an increased risk of MI[136] and perhaps stroke.[137] There are a number of potential reasons that these papers came to a different conclusion than our analysis and that of Wang and colleagues. The 2010 meta-analysis included 15 studies, only three of which met our criteria for inclusion. The other 12 studies were quite heterogeneous; some were small trials that contributed fewer than 20 events, another did not publish CVD events but supplied them for the meta-analysis,[138] and none were designed to examine CVD outcomes. Many lacked information on the adjudication of CVD events. The results of the meta-analysis were mainly driven by the three studies that were included in our review: ACS, RECORD, and CPPS; however, CPPS has not published CVD outcomes so we could not examine them. The results of pooled data from these three studies for any outcome must be interpreted cautiously because of their heterogeneity; ACS included healthy postmenopausal women, CPPS included men with a history of colorectal polyps, and RECORD included men and women with a history of fragility fracture.

The 2011 meta-analysis[137] incorporates a reanalysis of the WHI results, with some of the studies included in their first meta-analysis. The reanalysis of the WHI data selected only the women who were not using calcium or vitamin D supplements at baseline. Such post hoc subgroup analyses can be misleading. Also, in the 2010 meta-analysis, the authors state that the increase in CVD was seen only in the subgroup that was above the median intake of calcium at baseline; thus, it is not clear why one would expect that in WHI the harms of calcium supplementation would be seen in the lower-intake subgroup and not the higher-intake group. Furthermore, the WHI investigators conducted their own reanalysis of their trial results, stratified by baseline supplement use, and added the results of their large observational study.[112] They found no evidence of a harmful effect of calcium plus vitamin D on any CVD (or cancer) outcome in either the RCT or the cohort, both overall and in the subgroup not taking a supplement at baseline.

Other recent observational studies have also generated additional attention to the issue of harm from calcium supplementation. In 2013, Xiao and colleagues reported that calcium supplementation was associated with increased CVD deaths (RR, 1.20 [95% CI, 1.05 to 1.36]) in men but not women in the National Institutes of Health-AARP Diet and Health Study.[139] In 2012, Li and colleagues reported some evidence of lower MI risk with higher intake of dietary calcium but a higher risk of MI in those who reported taking a calcium supplement compared with those who did not (RR, 1.86 [95% CI, 1.17 to 2.96]).[140] Different results for dietary and supplemental calcium highlight the possibility of confounding in the supplement users. Overall, there is insufficient consistency in the recent observational studies to conclude that calcium supplementation is harmful, but the issue deserves additional study.

In general, the results of vitamin supplementation trials have been disappointing at best, despite having a solid mechanistic basis.[141] One explanation for this could be that the physiological systems affected by vitamins and other antioxidant supplements are complex, so the effects of superphysiological doses of only one or a few components are generally ineffective or actually do harm.[142] This possibility is compatible with the finding in this review that the best data for any salutary effects was for the two multivitamin trials, which used more physiologic doses of a wider variety of agents.

Limitations in the Body of Evidence

Despite the fact that about half of the U.S. population reports the use of vitamin and mineral supplements, at an annual cost of over $11 billion, there are few studies to support the effectiveness of such supplements in decreasing CVD, cancer, or mortality rates.

Published studies used a wide variety of supplements, in different doses and with different objectives and populations. Frequently, the data on CVD and cancer were derived from secondary analyses; only a few trials were designed to study the effects of a supplement on CVD or cancer. For most supplements, there were too few studies or too much clinical heterogeneity to allow for valid pooling of outcomes, limiting the power to detect effects. The individual studies often had small sample sizes, and because many were focused on specific outcomes (e.g., fractures), the samples were not generalizable to the typical primary care population. Even some large trials, such as PHS-II, have limited generalizability because of the recruitment methods. In PHS-II, all participants were male physicians and only 5 percent of those contacted participated. Another limitation is the short duration of most trials (around 5 years) relative to the long preclinical development of both CVD and cancer. The trials may have been simply too short to detect effects. On the other hand, it could be argued that 5 years of use is as long term as most of the general public will accept. We did not identify any studies examining the efficacy for CVD or cancer prevention of calcium in combination with magnesium, folic acid in combination with vitamin B_{12}, folic acid in combination with vitamin D_6, niacin, iron, magnesium, zinc and vitamins B_1, B_2, B_6, and B_{12}. We did not identify any studies examining the safety of iron supplementation and the few included trials that reported harms did so comprehensively.

Two additional design issues complicated our analysis. Several of the trials used factorial designs (2x2 or more complex combinations). Such designs are appealing because the ability to collapse across one intervention in analyzing another effectively doubles the sample size for each intervention. However, such analysis assumes that there is no biological interaction between the two interventions, and a formal statistical interaction test should be included in the first step of the analysis. If an interaction is present, then only the simple main effects may be examined (i.e., to examine factor A, only individuals in the factor B placebo condition may be used). Unfortunately, such tests for interaction are often overlooked, and even when done may be underpowered, unless the interaction effect is very large. Furthermore, in nutrition trials many nutrients would be expected to interact biologically (e.g., two antioxidant supplements). Most of the factorial supplement studies included in this report reported on interaction tests and found none (SELECT was an exception, finding that cosupplementation with selenium erased the modest increased risk of prostate cancer seen in the vitamin E only group).[143] A discussion of the power issue was rare. Given the presumed biology behind these supplements, the lack of significant interactions supports the likelihood of little or no true effect.

A related design limitation is the inflation of type I error introduced by multiple testing. As noted, most of the studies were not designed to test hypotheses about CVD and cancer prevention. Secondary analyses, especially when subgroups are involved, can be problematic in general, and when they include tests for treatment differences on multiple outcomes, the likelihood of a type I error increases. For example, several studies examined site-specific cancer incidence as secondary analyses, without any correction of the significance values for the number of tests.

Most of the trials were conducted in populations of European ancestry, so the results may not be generalizable to other race/ethnicity groups. While there is no a priori reason to believe that the biology that these supplements might affect differs across racial/ethnic groups, the differences in other risk factors for CVD and cancer (e.g., nutritional, physical activity, or socioeconomic circumstances) among these groups in the United States could affect the outcomes.

Limitations in Our Approach

While this systematic review considered a broad range of studies and supplements, it was also focused in important ways. We considered only primary prevention interventions in generally healthy people, excluding secondary prevention trials aimed only at the disease in question and tertiary prevention or treatment studies. In some cases, however, we included secondary prevention studies if the supplement was also intended to prevent other relevant disease that was not present at baseline, mortality, or both (e.g., SCPS examined the efficacy of supplementation to prevent other cancers in patients with a previous BCC or SCC). We also excluded studies in which participants had active CVD and/or cancer at baseline.

We excluded studies of individuals with nutritional deficiencies. This criterion eliminated the Linxian study, a large multivitamin trial in China that included individuals with baseline nutritional deficiency.[144] The Linxian study, which supports the use of multivitamin supplements, has been included in previous reviews of this topic, as have secondary prevention trials. We also focused on supplement doses that were below the recommended upper limit (or so-called "nutritional doses"), so our results do not pertain to high-dose vitamin or mineral therapy, which in any case should be treated as a pharmacological intervention.

We also excluded studies that did not include CVD, cancer, or all-cause mortality as an a priori aim of the study (whether primary or secondary). The purpose of this exclusion criterion was to focus on studies designed to assess the questions posed for this review. As noted previously, post hoc analyses of secondary outcomes are more subject to biased or chance findings, but many other systematic reviews and meta-analyses have included such studies in their assessment of outcomes. Note that if we included a trial designed to answer one of the outcomes, we also report analyses of secondary outcomes as long as there was some indication that these analyses were planned at baseline.

Our definition of a multivitamin as containing three or more supplements was arbitrary. Even this inclusive definition included only two trials for efficacy. However, those two trials studied very different supplements: five components in SU.VI.MAX. and 32 in PHS-II. Since only the former trial included women, it could be argued that there are no data on a "true" multivitamin in women. The SU.VI.MAX supplement included agents expected to improve both inflammation and oxidative stress and showed benefit for cancer incidence in men, matching the PHS-II results, so the importance of this difference is debatable.

The number of supplements included in this review also presented a challenge for reporting on harms. A very large number of adverse events may be included, especially from observational studies, where the unexposed group may not be comparable with the exposed group. Instead we took a narrower approach by examining harms in the randomized trials primarily. We also limited the analysis of mortality results to RCTs.

This is a review of randomized clinical trials, a design that was created primarily to evaluate drug therapy. It can be argued that the typical implementation of this design is not ideally suited to evaluating nutrients rather than drugs.[145] In placebo-controlled trials of medications, the control group is not exposed to the medication. In a nutrient supplementation study, however, the control group is exposed to some level of the agent under study. The question is different: is an optimal level of exposure to the nutrient better than the usual level? To conduct such a study implies that both the usual level of exposure and the optimal level are known. Different levels of exposure are also possible in drug trials, of course, but most drug RCTs for efficacy are preceded by dosing studies that define the "best" dose. Thus the threat of an insufficient difference between the exposure in the treatment and control groups is greater for a nutrient study. Lappe and Heaney cite the example of the WHI calcium and vitamin D study.[145] When that study was designed, average calcium intake was about half of what was observed in the actual control group; the subsequent increase in average calcium intake narrowed the dose difference between groups and may have created a control group that had already achieved all the benefit possible from calcium intake. Similarly, the dose of vitamin D in WHI was lower than many now think is necessary to achieve adequate blood levels, although there is still great uncertainty about the optimal level. We are not arguing that RCTs of nutritional supplements are invalid; such studies do indeed test the effects of the supplement versus no supplement, but changes in average intake (in the control group) are an additional threat to these studies compared with drug studies.

Finally, by focusing our review on nutrient supplementation to improve nutritional status in generally replete adults, the targeted use of nutrients in deficient or higher-risk individuals was not completely addressed. Our results are consistent with potential benefit of higher doses in those with suboptimal nutrient status. For example, Lappe and colleagues' vitamin D and calcium study found some evidence of a benefit on cancer using a relatively high dose of vitamin D (1,000 IU/d) in a population known to have low average vitamin D levels.[109] Similarly, the effects of selenium seen in the NPC study[89] was confined to participants with low baseline selenium levels.

Applicability

The purpose of this review was to describe the evidence of benefit on cancer and CVD morbidity and mortality from vitamin and mineral supplementation in generally healthy, nutritionally-replete adults. Only two included trials directly addressed these questions in the intended population. One used a more typical multiple vitamin and mineral formulation but was limited to predominately white male physicians[50] and the other recruited a general population but used a supplement with just five ingredients.[49] Thus, even these studies have somewhat limited applicability in underrepresenting women and nonEuropean populations. Since SU.VI.MAX found an effect only in men, the lack of another study in women is particularly limiting.

All of the other trials included in the review used only one or two nutrients, with limited numbers of studies for each. Few of these studies were designed to test effects on cancer or CVD endpoints, and many enrolled selected populations, populations with unrelated disease such as cataracts (we excluded secondary prevention studies), or smokers. Most of the calcium and vitamin D studies were directed at fracture prevention. The applicability of these targeted populations to the general population is thus limited, though not absent, particularly when viewed together.

In addition, the majority of included studies specifically recruited middle-aged (45 to 64 years) and older adults (≥65 years); therefore, the body of evidence included in this review is most applicable to these populations. Children and younger adults are not represented in these studies. With older age comes a greater risk for CVD, cancer, and mortality. As a result, we can expect higher numbers of these events in older age groups and any subgroup analyses that show an increase in these outcomes with older age should be interpreted cautiously. Correspondingly, one might expect a potentially larger benefit in preventing these health outcomes with vitamin and/or mineral supplementation in older populations who may be less nutritionally replete than younger age groups. When examined in post hoc subgroup analyses, some studies found small but statistically significant differences between older and younger subgroups on outcomes,[57] but overall, there were few differences by age within studies.

Future Research

Our review highlights a series of evidence gaps. Despite there being two relatively large trials examining the efficacy of a multivitamin in the primary prevention of CVD and cancer in a general population, population selection and potential sex-specific findings limit the applicability of their results. Clearly, there is a large knowledge gap on the effects of multivitamins on CVD, cancer, and many other endpoints. To study this question, future trials should recruit from a general population with representation of multiple minority groups and both sexes, employ a multivitamin that is reasonably similar to the popular brands in the current market, and include enough participants to provide adequate power to detect benefits and harms. This is a tall order, and any such study would still face difficulties. Agreement on the content of the multivitamin would likely be difficult to achieve, so the results of the trial might be dismissed by observers who felt that an important ingredient was omitted. The wide availability of multivitamins could result in significant crossover. The large number of participants and long followup needed would result in an expensive trial. It is doubtful that any multivitamin manufacturer would see the wisdom of supporting such a trial, making it more difficult to fund. Still, the U.S public is devoting significant resources to multivitamins, so such a trial could have significant public health benefit, whatever the outcome.

Despite its limitations, the current literature on single or paired vitamins and minerals is sufficient to discourage additional studies of beta-carotene; vitamins A, C, or E; and folic acid in general populations or especially among those at high risk of the endpoint and not deficient in the nutrient to be supplemented. Future studies of selenium would need to clearly separate individuals with adequate and low baseline selenium levels. Vitamin D and calcium are currently indicated for fracture prevention but their effects on other endpoints are unclear. Despite their close relationship on bone health, future studies would be better if vitamin D and calcium were studied separately, as they may have different effects; in particular, calcium alone may have harmful effects on CVD. At least six studies of vitamin D alone are in process; no ongoing study of calcium alone was identified. Such studies should include fracture outcomes as well, since it will be necessary to balance benefits on bone health against any harms for CVD, cancer, or mortality.

The points made by Lappe and Heaney in their recent article are relevant to additional studies of nutritional supplements.[145] Unlike drug studies, control groups in nutrient studies are also exposed to the agent under investigation. Careful thought needs to be given to the biology of the nutrient and current understanding of average and presumed optimal levels. A broad diet that includes adequate plant-based foods is likely to supply sufficient nutrients for health in the general population. Supplements may be warranted if the actual diet strays from the natural diet or other factors come into play (e.g., reduced sun exposure lowering vitamin D levels). Measurement of exposure in both treatment and control groups would likely help with the interpretation of the diet, and some supplements may be reserved for individuals with known low levels, when these can be measured. Controlled clinical trials are indicated when there is equipoise toward the benefits and harms of the agent to be studied; this point can be hard to discern (and may be fleeting) for any study, but for nutrient supplements it may be particularly difficult to define when a trial is needed. Sometimes trials should be delayed if the biological understanding of a nutrient's role in health is evolving.

We did not identify any studies examining the efficacy for CVD or cancer prevention of calcium in combination with magnesium, folic acid in combination with vitamin B_{12}, folic acid in combination with vitamin B_6, niacin, iron, magnesium, zinc, and vitamins B_1, B_2, B_6, and B_{12}. We did not identify any studies examining the safety of iron supplementation. Future studies of these nutrients may be useful, keeping in mind the cautions of the previous paragraph.

We identified 11 relevant ongoing trials in healthy adults through national and international clinical trial registries. Each study listed cancer, CVD, mortality, or harms as primary or secondary outcomes (**Appendix C**). These trials are evaluating single or paired vitamins and minerals, including vitamin D alone or in combination with calcium (n=8), selenium with or without vitamin E (n=2), and vitamin C (n=1). We did not identify any published ongoing studies of multivitamins or other supplements in children, so this could be an important area for future research.

Conclusions

For most of the supplements addressed in this report, we found no evidence of an effect of nutritional doses on CVD, cancer, or mortality in healthy individuals with a generally adequate diet. In most cases there are insufficient data to draw any conclusion. One exception in this report are the two multivitamin studies, SU.VI.MAX and PHS-II, which both found lower overall cancer incidence in men. While these trials were both methodologically rated as good, the lack of effect (and limited data) on women in SU.VI.MAX, the modest effect in men in both trials, and the lack of any effect in either study on CVD makes it difficult to recommend that supplementation with any vitamin will provide protection against CVD or cancer. Another exception are the two beta-carotene trials among individuals at high risk for lung cancer, which found a statistically significant increased risk of developing and dying from lung cancer.

Adequate dietary intake of calcium and vitamin D is necessary for bone health and to prevent osteoporosis and fracture.[8] Supplementation with calcium and vitamin D have long been advocated to insure adequate intake, especially in postmenopausal women. However, in February

2013 the USPSTF recommended against supplementation with 400 IU or less of vitamin D or 1,000 mg or less of calcium for fracture prevention.[146] In addition, existing data are compatible with the possibility that vitamin D and calcium have different effects on CVD and all-cause mortality. Future studies of calcium and vitamin D directed at CVD prevention should separate the effects of these two nutrients, and careful attention to dose is needed.

Few harms were identified in the included trials and observational cohort studies. There was no consistent pattern within each nutrient group and few people discontinued vitamin use due to adverse effects. This finding is consistent with the use of nutrients only within RDA amounts. The one exception is the association of beta-carotene supplements with increased lung cancer in trials of individuals exposed to tobacco smoke or asbestos. This finding, however, was not seen in other beta-carotene trials not restricted to high-risk individuals.

References

1. U.S. Preventive Services Task Force. Routine vitamin supplementation to prevent cancer and cardiovascular disease: recommendations and rationale. *Ann Intern Med.* 2003;139(1):51-5. PMID: 12834319.
2. Otten JJ, Hellwig JP, Meyers LD (eds). Dietary Reference Intakes: The Essential Guide to Nutrient Requirements. Washington, DC: National Academies Press; 2006.
3. Institute of Medicine. Dietary Reference Intakes for Calcium, Phosphorous, Magnesium, Vitamin D, and Fluoride. Washington, DC: National Academy Press; 1997.
4. Institute of Medicine. Dietary Reference Intakes for Thiamin, Riboflavin, Niacin, Vitamin B6, Folate, Vitamin B12, Pantothenic Acide, Biotin, and Choline. Washington, DC: National Academies Press; 1998.
5. Institute of Medicine. Dietary reference Intakes for Vitamin C, Vitamin E, Selenium, and Carotenoids. Washington, DC: National Academies Press; 2000.
6. Institute of Medicine. Dietary Reference Intakes for Vitamin A, Vitamin K, Arsenic, Boron, Chromium, Copper, Iodine, Iron, Manganese, Molybdenum, Nickel, Silicon, Vanadium, and Zinc. Washington, DC: National Academies Press; 2001.
7. Institute of Medicine. Dietary Reference Intakes for Water, Potassium, Sodium, Chloride, and Sulfate. Washington, DC: National Academies Press; 2005.
8. Institute of Medicine. Dietary Reference Intakes for Calcium and Vitamin D. Washington, DC: National Academies Press; 2011.
9. Radimer K, Bindewald B, Hughes J, et al. Dietary supplement use by US adults: data from the National Health and Nutrition Examination Survey, 1999-2000. *Am J Epidemiol.* 2004;160(4):339-49. PMID: 15286019.
10. Bailey RL, Gahche JJ, Lentino CV, et al. Dietary supplement use in the United States, 2003-2006. *J Nutr.* 2011;141(2):261-6. PMID: 21178089.
11. Gahche J, Bailey R, Burt V, et al. Dietary supplement use among U.S. adults has increased since NHANES III (1988-1994). *NCHS Data Brief.* 2011;(61):1-8. PMID: 21592424.
12. Nutrition Business Journal. NBJ's Supplement Business Report: An Analysis of Markets, Trends, Competition and Strategy in the U.S. Dietary Supplement Industry. New York: Penton Media; 2011.
13. Dwyer J. Why Do Americans Use Dietary Supplements? Motivation for Dietary Supplement Use. American Dietetic Association Food and Nutrition Conference and Expo; Oct 24, 2005; St. Louis, MO.
14. Dickinson A, Boyon N, Shao A. Physicians and nurses use and recommend dietary supplements: report of a survey. *Nutr J.* 2009;8:29. PMID: 19570197.
15. Dickinson A, Shao A, Boyon N, et al. Use of dietary supplements by cardiologists, dermatologists and orthopedists: report of a survey. *Nutr J.* 2011;10:20. PMID: 21371318.
16. Dickinson A, Bonci L, Boyon N, et al. Dietitians use and recommend dietary supplements: report of a survey. *Nutr J.* 2012;11:14. PMID: 22416673.
17. Go AS, Mozaffarian D, Roger VL, et al. Heart disease and stroke statistics—2013 update: a report from the American Heart Association. *Circulation.* 2013;127(1):e6-245. PMID: 23239837.

18. Fang J, Shaw KM, Keenan NL. Prevalence of coronary heart disease: United States, 2006-2010. *MMWR Morb Mortal Wkly Rep*. 2011;60(40):1377-81.
19. Centers for Disease Control and Prevention. Leading Causes of Death. Atlanta: Centers for Disease Control and Prevention; 2012. Accessed at http://www.cdc.gov/nchs/fastats/lcod.htm/ on 7 October 2013.
20. Surveillance Epidemiology and End Results. Cancer Stat Fact Sheets. Bethesda, MD: National Cancer Institute; 2012. Accessed at http://seer.cancer.gov/statfacts on 7 October 2013.
21. Yusuf S, Hawken S, Ounpuu S, et al. Effect of potentially modifiable risk factors associated with myocardial infarction in 52 countries (the INTERHEART study): case-control study. *Lancet*. 2004;364(9438):937-52. PMID: 15364185.
22. Geffken DF, Cushman M, Burke GL, et al. Association between physical activity and markers of inflammation in a healthy elderly population. *Am J Epidemiol*. 2001;153(3):242-50. PMID: 11157411.
23. Libby P, Ridker PM, Hansson GK. Progress and challenges in translating the biology of atherosclerosis. *Nature*. 2011;473(7347):317-25. PMID: 21593864.
24. Steinberg D, Parthasarathy S, Carew TE, et al. Beyond cholesterol. Modifications of low-density lipoprotein that increase its atherogenicity. *N Engl J Med*. 1989;320(14):915-24. PMID: 2648148.
25. Loft S, Poulsen HE. Cancer risk and oxidative DNA damage in man. *J Mol Med (Berl)*. 1996;74(6):297-312. PMID: 8862511.
26. Davis CD, Uthus EO. DNA methylation, cancer susceptibility, and nutrient interactions. *Exp Biol Med (Maywood)*. 2004;229(10):988-95. PMID: 15522834.
27. Das PM, Singal R. DNA methylation and cancer. *J Clin Oncol*. 2004;22(22):4632-42. PMID: 15542813.
28. Robinson K (ed). Homocysteine and Vascular Disease. Norwell, MA: Kluwer Academic Publishers; 2000.
29. Edgar RM, Stephen J, Roberto PB, et al. Meta-analysis of folic acid supplementation trials on risk of cardiovascular disease and risk interaction with baseline homocysteine levels. *Am J Cardiology*. 2010;106(517):527. PMID: 20691310.
30. Spence JD, Stampfer MJ. Understanding the complexity of homocysteine lowering with vitamins: the potential role of subgroup analyses. *JAMA*. 2011;306(23):2610-1. PMID: 22187282.
31. Tosetti F, Ferrari N, De Flora S, et al. Angioprevention: angiogenesis is a common and key target for cancer chemopreventive agents. *FASEB J*. 2002;16(1):2-14. PMID: 11772931.
32. Ashino H, Shimamura M, Nakajima H, et al. Novel function of ascorbic acid as an angiostatic factor. *Angiogenesis*. 2003;6(4):259-69. PMID: 15166494.
33. Reifen R. Vitamin A as an anti-inflammatory agent. *Proc Nutr Soc*. 2002;61(3):397-400. PMID: 12230799.
34. Bogden JD. Influence of zinc on immunity in the elderly. *J Nutr Health Aging*. 2004;8(1):48-54. PMID: 14730367.
35. Villamor E, Fawzi WW. Effects of vitamin A supplementation on immune responses and correlation with clinical outcomes. *Clin Microbiol Rev*. 2005;18(3):446-64. PMID: 16020684.

36. Huang HY, Berndt S, Helzlsouer KJ. Vitamin E as a cancer chemopreventive agent. In: Kelloff GJ, Hawk ET, Sigman CC (eds). Cancer Chemoprevention. Volume 1: Promising Cancer Chemopreventive Agents. New Jersey: Humana Press; 2004.
37. Morris CD, Carson S. Routine Vitamin Supplementation to Prevent Cardiovascular Disease: A Summary of the Evidence for the U.S. Preventive Services Task Force. AHRQ Publication No. 03-523B. Rockville, MD: Agency for Healthcare Research and Quality; 2003.
38. Ritenbaugh C, Streit K, Helfand M. Routine Vitamin Supplementation to Prevent Cancer: A Summary of Evidence From Randomized, Controlled Trials for the U.S. Preventive Services Task Force. AHRQ Publication No. 03-523C. Rockville, MD: Agency for Healthcare Research and Quality; 2003.
39. Atkins D, Shetty P. Routine Vitamin Supplementation to Prevent Cancer: Update of the Evidence From Randomized, Controlled Trials, 1999-2002. AHRQ Publication No. 03-523D. Rockville, MD: Agency for Healthcare Research and Quality; 2003.
40. Huang HY, Caballero B, Chang S, et al. Multivitamin/Mineral Supplements and Prevention of Chronic Disease. AHRQ Publication No. 139. Rockville, MD: Agency for Healthcare Research and Quality; 2006.
41. Gordis L. Epidemiology. Philadelphia: Saunders Elsevier; 2009.
42. Chou R, Aronson N, Atkins D, et al. AHRQ series paper 4: assessing harms when comparing medical interventions: AHRQ and the Effective Health Care Program. *J Clin Epidemiol*. 2010;63(5):502-12. PMID: 18823754.
43. Human Development Report 2011. Sustainability and Equity: A Better Future for All. New York: United Nations Development Programme; 2011.
44. U.S. Preventive Services Task Force. Procedure Manual. AHRQ Publication No. 08-05118-EF. Rockville, MD: Agency for Healthcare Research and Quality; 2008.
45. National Institute for Health and Clinical Excellence. The Guidelines Manual. London: National Institute for Health and Clinical Excellence; 2006.
46. Bradburn MJ, Deeks JJ, Altman DG. Metan-a command for meta-analysis in Stata. In: Sterne JA (ed). Meta-Analysis in Stata: An Updated Collection From the Stata Journal. College Station, TX: Stata Press; 1998. p. 3-28.
47. Fu R, Gartlehner G, Grant M, et al. Conducting quantitative synthesis when comparing medical interventions: AHRQ and the Effective Health Care Program. *J Clin Epidemiol*. 2011;64(11):1187-97. PMID: 21477993.
48. DerSimonian R, Laird N. Meta-analysis in clinical trials. *Control Clin Trials*. 1986;7(3):177-88. PMID: 3802833.
49. Hercberg S, Galan P, Preziosi P, et al. The SU.VI.MAX study: a randomized, placebo-controlled trial of the health effects of antioxidant vitamins and minerals. *Arch Intern Med*. 2004;164(21):2335-42. PMID: 15557412.
50. Gaziano J, Sesso HD, Christen HJ, et al. Multivitamins in the prevention of cancer in men: the Physicians' Health Study II randomized controlled trial. *JAMA*. 2012;308(18):1871-80. PMID: 23162860.
51. Chylack LT Jr, Brown NP, Bron A, et al. The Roche European American Cataract Trial (REACT): a randomized clinical trial to investigate the efficacy of an oral antioxidant micronutrient mixture to slow progression of age-related cataract. *Ophthalmic Epidemiol*. 2002;9(1):49-80. PMID: 11815895.

52. Graat JM, Schouten EG, Kok FJ. Effect of daily vitamin E and multivitamin-mineral supplementation on acute respiratory tract infections in elderly persons: a randomized controlled trial. *JAMA*. 2002;288(6):715-21. PMID: 12169075.
53. Feskanich D, Singh V, Willett WC, et al. Vitamin A intake and hip fractures among postmenopausal women. *JAMA*. 2002;287(1):47-54. PMID: 11754708.
54. Hercberg S, Galan P, Preziosi P, et al. Background and rationale behind the SU.VI.MAX study, a prevention trial using nutritional doses of a combination of antioxidant vitamins and minerals to reduce cardiovascular diseases and cancers. *Int J Vitam Nutr Res*. 1998;68(1):3-20. PMID: 9503043.
55. Meyer F, Galan P, Douville P, et al. Antioxidant vitamin and mineral supplementation and prostate cancer prevention in the SU.VI.MAX trial. *Int J Cancer*. 2005;116(2):182-6. PMID: 15800922.
56. Hercberg S, Kesse-Guyot E, Druesne-Pecollo N, et al. Incidence of cancers, ischemic cardiovascular diseases and mortality during 5-year follow-up after stopping antioxidant vitamins and minerals supplements: a postintervention follow-up in the SU.VI.MAX study. *Int J Cancer*. 2010;127(8):1875-81. PMID: 20104528.
57. Sesso HD, Christen WG, Bubes V, et al. Multivitamins in the prevention of cardiovascular disease in men: the Physicians' Health Study II randomized controlled trial. *JAMA*. 2012;308(17):1751-60. PMID: 23117775.
58. Hercberg S, Ezzedine K, Guinot C, et al. Antioxidant supplementation increases the risk of skin cancers in women but not in men. *J Nutr*. 2007;137(9):2098-105. PMID: 17709449.
59. Alpha-Tocopherol Beta Carotene Cancer Prevention Study Group. The effect of vitamin E and beta carotene on the incidence of lung cancer and other cancers in male smokers. *N Engl J Med*. 1994;330(15):1029-35. PMID: 8127329.
60. Omenn GS, Goodman GE, Thornquist MD, et al. Effects of a combination of beta carotene and vitamin A on lung cancer and cardiovascular disease. *N Engl J Med*. 1996;334(18):1150-5. PMID: 8602180.
61. Hennekens CH, Buring JE, Manson JE, et al. Lack of effect of long-term supplementation with beta carotene on the incidence of malignant neoplasms and cardiovascular disease. *N Engl J Med*. 1996;334(18):1145-9. PMID: 8602179.
62. Lee IM, Cook NR, Manson JE, et al. Beta-carotene supplementation and incidence of cancer and cardiovascular disease: the Women's Health Study. *J Natl Cancer Inst*. 1999;91(24):2102-6. PMID: 10601381.
63. Greenberg ER, Baron JA, Stukel TA, et al; Skin Cancer Prevention Study Group. A clinical trial of beta carotene to prevent basal-cell and squamous-cell cancers of the skin. *N Engl J Med*. 1990;323(12):789-95. PMID: 2202901.
64. Green A, Williams G, Neale R, et al. Daily sunscreen application and betacarotene supplementation in prevention of basal-cell and squamous-cell carcinomas of the skin: a randomised controlled trial. *Lancet*. 1999;354(9180):723-9. PMID: 10475183.
65. Liu S, Ajani U, Chae C, et al. Long-term beta-carotene supplementation and risk of type 2 diabetes mellitus: a randomized controlled trial. *JAMA*. 1999;282(11):1073-5. PMID: 10493207.
66. Kataja-Tuomola M, Sundell JR, Mannisto S, et al. Effect of alpha-tocopherol and beta-carotene supplementation on the incidence of type 2 diabetes. *Diabetologia*. 2008;51(1):47-53. PMID: 17994292.

67. Omenn GS, Goodman GE, Thornquist MD, et al. Risk factors for lung cancer and for intervention effects in CARET, the Beta-Carotene and Retinol Efficacy Trial. *J Natl Cancer Inst*. 1996;88(21):1550-9. PMID: 8901853.
68. Cook NR, Le IM, Manson JE, et al. Effects of beta-carotene supplementation on cancer incidence by baseline characteristics in the Physicians' Health Study (United States). *Cancer Causes Control*. 2000;11(7):617-26. PMID: 10977106.
69. Rautalahti MT, Virtamo JR, Taylor PR, et al. The effects of supplementation with alpha-tocopherol and beta-carotene on the incidence and mortality of carcinoma of the pancreas in a randomized, controlled trial. *Cancer*. 1999;86(1):37-42. PMID: 10391561.
70. Malila N, Taylor PR, Virtanen MJ, et al. Effects of alpha-tocopherol and beta-carotene supplementation on gastric cancer incidence in male smokers (ATBC Study, Finland). *Cancer Causes Control*. 2002;13(7):617-23. PMID: 12296509.
71. Virtamo J, Edwards BK, Virtanen M, et al. Effects of supplemental alpha-tocopherol and beta-carotene on urinary tract cancer: incidence and mortality in a controlled trial (Finland). *Cancer Causes Control*. 2000;11(10):933-9. PMID: 11142528.
72. Wright ME, Virtamo J, Hartman AM, et al. Effects of alpha-tocopherol and beta-carotene supplementation on upper aerodigestive tract cancers in a large, randomized controlled trial. *Cancer*. 2007;109(5):891-8. PMID: 17265529.
73. Virtamo J, Pietinen P, Huttunen JK, et al. Incidence of cancer and mortality following alpha-tocopherol and beta-carotene supplementation: a postintervention follow-up. *JAMA*. 2003;290(4):476-85. PMID: 12876090.
74. Goodman GE, Thornquist MD, Balmes J, et al. The Beta-Carotene and Retinol Efficacy Trial: incidence of lung cancer and cardiovascular disease mortality during 6-year follow-up after stopping beta-carotene and retinol supplements. *J Natl Cancer Inst*. 2004;96(23):1743-50. PMID: 15572756.
75. Greenberg ER, Baron JA, Karagas MR, et al. Mortality associated with low plasma concentration of beta carotene and the effect of oral supplementation. *JAMA*. 1996;275(9):699-703. PMID: 8594267.
76. Heinonen OP, Albanes D, Virtamo J, et al. Prostate cancer and supplementation with alpha-tocopherol and beta-carotene: incidence and mortality in a controlled trial. *J Natl Cancer Inst*. 1998;90(6):440-6. PMID: 9521168.
77. Albanes D, Malila N, Taylor PR, et al. Effects of supplemental alpha-tocopherol and beta-carotene on colorectal cancer: results from a controlled trial (Finland). *Cancer Causes Control*. 2000;11(3):197-205. PMID: 10782653.
78. Hemila H, Virtamo J, Albanes D, et al. Vitamin E and beta-carotene supplementation and hospital-treated pneumonia incidence in male smokers. *Chest*. 2004;125(2):557-65. PMID: 14769738.
79. Salonen JT, Nyyssonen K, Salonen R, et al. Antioxidant Supplementation in Atherosclerosis Prevention (ASAP) study: a randomized trial of the effect of vitamins E and C on 3-year progression of carotid atherosclerosis. *J Intern Med*. 2000;248(5):377-86. PMID: 11123502.
80. Sesso HD, Buring JE, Christen WG, et al. Vitamins E and C in the prevention of cardiovascular disease in men: the Physicians' Health Study II randomized controlled trial. *JAMA*. 2008;300(18):2123-33. PMID: 18997197.

81. Lee IM, Cook NR, Gaziano JM, et al. Vitamin E in the primary prevention of cardiovascular disease and cancer: the Women's Health Study: a randomized controlled trial. *JAMA*. 2005;294(1):56-65. PMID: 15998891.
82. Lippman SM, Klein EA, Goodman PJ, et al. Effect of selenium and vitamin E on risk of prostate cancer and other cancers: the Selenium and Vitamin E Cancer Prevention Trial (SELECT). *JAMA*. 2009;301(1):39-51. PMID: 19066370.
83. Gaziano JM, Glynn RJ, Christen WG, et al. Vitamins E and C in the prevention of prostate and total cancer in men: the Physicians' Health Study II randomized controlled trial. *JAMA*. 2009;301(1):52-62. PMID: 19066368.
84. Ridker PM, Cook NR, Lee IM, et al. A randomized trial of low-dose aspirin in the primary prevention of cardiovascular disease in women: editorial comment. *Obstet Gynecol Surv*. 2005;60(8):519-21. PMID: 15753114.
85. Steering Committee of the Physicians' Health Study Research Group. Final report on the aspirin component of the ongoing Physicians' Health Study. *N Engl J Med*. 1989;321(3):129-35. PMID: 2664509.
86. Lotan Y, Goodman P, Youssef R, et al. Evaluation of vitamin E and selenium supplementation on the prevention of bladder cancer in SWOG coordinated select. *J Urol*. 2012;187(6):2005-10. PMID: 22498220.
87. Hemila H, Kaprio J. Vitamin E supplementation and pneumonia risk in males who initiated smoking at an early age: effect modification by body weight and dietary vitamin C. *Nutr J*. 2008;7:33. PMID: 19019244.
88. Hemila H, Kaprio J. Subgroup analysis of large trials can guide further research: a case study of vitamin E and pneumonia. *Clin Epidemiol*. 2011;3(1):51-9. PMID: 21386974.
89. Clark LC, Combs GF Jr, Turnbull BW, et al; Nutritional Prevention of Cancer Study Group. Effects of selenium supplementation for cancer prevention in patients with carcinoma of the skin. A randomized controlled trial. *JAMA*. 1996;276(24):1957-63. PMID: 8971064.
90. Duffield-Lillico AJ, Reid ME, Turnbull BW, et al. Baseline characteristics and the effect of selenium supplementation on cancer incidence in a randomized clinical trial: a summary report of the Nutritional Prevention of Cancer Trial. *Cancer Epidemiol Biomarkers Prev*. 2002;11(7):630-9. PMID: 12101110.
91. Rayman MP, Blundell-Pound G, Pastor-Barriuso R, et al. A randomized trial of selenium supplementation and risk of type-2 diabetes, as assessed by plasma adiponectin. *PLoS One*. 2012;7(9):e45269. PMID: 16636212.
92. Combs GF Jr, Clark LC, Turnbull BW. Reduction of cancer mortality and incidence by selenium supplementation. *Med Klin (Munich)*. 1997;92(Suppl 3):42-5. PMID: 9342915.
93. Clark LC, Dalkin B, Krongrad A, et al. Decreased incidence of prostate cancer with selenium supplementation: results of a double-blind cancer prevention trial. *Br J Urol*. 1998;81(5):730-4. PMID: 9634050.
94. Reid ME, Duffield-Lillico AJ, Garland L, et al. Selenium supplementation and lung cancer incidence: an update of the nutritional prevention of cancer trial. *Cancer Epidemiol Biomarkers Prev*. 2002;11(11):1285-91. PMID: 12433704.
95. Duffield-Lillico AJ, Dalkin BL, Reid ME, et al. Selenium supplementation, baseline plasma selenium status and incidence of prostate cancer: an analysis of the complete treatment period of the Nutritional Prevention of Cancer Trial. *BJU Int*. 2003;91(7):608-12. PMID: 12699469.

96. Lim LS, Harnack LJ, Lazovich D, et al. Vitamin A intake and the risk of hip fracture in postmenopausal women: the Iowa Women's Health Study. *Osteoporos Int.* 2004;15(7):552-9. PMID: 14760518.
97. Moon TE, Levine N, Cartmel B, et al; Southwest Skin Cancer Prevention Study Group. Effect of retinol in preventing squamous cell skin cancer in moderate-risk subjects: a randomized, double-blind, controlled trial. *Cancer Epidemiol Biomarkers Prev.* 1997;6(11):949-56. PMID: 9367069.
98. Levine N, Moon TE, Cartmel B, et al; Southwest Skin Cancer Prevention Study Group. Trial of retinol and isotretinoin in skin cancer prevention: a randomized, double-blind, controlled trial. *Cancer Epidemiol Biomarkers Prev.* 1997;6(11):957-61. PMID: 9367070.
99. Melhus H, Michaelsson K, Kindmark A, et al. Excessive dietary intake of vitamin A is associated with reduced bone mineral density and increased risk for hip fracture. *Ann Intern Med.* 1998;129(10):770-8. PMID: 9841582.
100. Promislow JH, Goodman-Gruen D, Slymen DJ, et al. Retinol intake and bone mineral density in the elderly: the Rancho Bernardo Study. *J Bone Miner Res.* 2002;17(8):1349-58. PMID: 12162487.
101. Cole BF, Baron JA, Sandler RS, et al. Folic acid for the prevention of colorectal adenomas: a randomized clinical trial. *JAMA.* 2007;297(21):2351-9. PMID: 17551129.
102. Figueiredo JC, Grau MV, Haile RW, et al. Folic acid and risk of prostate cancer: results from a randomized clinical trial. *J Natl Cancer Inst.* 2009;101(6):432-5. PMID: 19276452.
103. Avenell A, MacLennan GS, Jenkinson DJ, et al. Long-term follow-up for mortality and cancer in a randomized placebo-controlled trial of vitamin D(3) and/or calcium (RECORD trial). *J Clin Endocrinol Metab.* 2012;97(2):614-22. PMID: 22112804.
104. Trivedi DP, Doll R, Khaw KT. Effect of four monthly oral vitamin D3 (cholecalciferol) supplementation on fractures and mortality in men and women living in the community: randomised double blind controlled trial. *BMJ.* 2003;326(7387):469. PMID: 12609940.
105. Dean AJ, Bellgrove MA, Hall T, et al. Effects of vitamin D supplementation on cognitive and emotional functioning in young adults—a randomised controlled trial. *PLoS One.* 2011;6(11):e25966. PMID: 22073146.
106. Ford JA, MacLennan G, Bolland MJ, et al. Vitamin D supplementation prevents cardiac failure; MRC record trial analysis, systematic review and meta-analysis. *Circulation.* 2012;126:A18397.
107. Grant AM, Avenell A, Campbell MK, et al. Oral vitamin D3 and calcium for secondary prevention of low-trauma fractures in elderly people (Randomised Evaluation of Calcium or Vitamin D, RECORD): a randomised placebo-controlled trial. *Lancet.* 2005;365(9471):1621-8. PMID: 15885294.
108. Wactawski-Wende J, Kotchen JM, Anderson GL, et al. Calcium plus vitamin D supplementation and the risk of colorectal cancer. *N Engl J Med.* 2006;354(7):684-96. PMID: 16481636.
109. Lappe JM, Travers-Gustafson D, Davies KM, et al. Vitamin D and calcium supplementation reduces cancer risk: results of a randomized trial. *Am J Clin Nutr.* 2007;85(6):1586-91. PMID: 17556697.

110. de Boer I, Tinker LF, Connelly S, et al. Calcium plus vitamin D supplementation and the risk of incident diabetes in the Women's Health Initiative. *Diabetes Care.* 2008;31(4):701-7. PMID: 18235052.
111. Bolland MJ, Grey A, Gamble GD, et al. Calcium and vitamin D supplements and health outcomes: a reanalysis of the Women's Health Initiative (WHI) limited-access data set. *Am J Clin Nutr.* 2011;94(4):1144-9. PMID: 21880848.
112. Prentice RL, Pettinger MB, Jackson RD, et al. Health risks and benefits from calcium and vitamin D supplementation: Women's Health Initiative clinical trial and cohort study. *Osteoporos Int.* 2013;24(2):567-80. PMID: 23208074.
113. Bolland MJ, Barber PA, Doughty RN, et al. Vascular events in healthy older women receiving calcium supplementation: randomised controlled trial. *BMJ.* 2008;336(7638):262-6. PMID: 18198394.
114. Baron JA, Beach M, Wallace K, et al. Risk of prostate cancer in a randomized clinical trial of calcium supplementation. *Cancer Epidemiol Biomarkers Prev.* 2005;14(3):586-9. PMID: 15767334.
115. Reid IR, Mason B, Horne A, et al. Randomized controlled trial of calcium in healthy older women. *Am J Med.* 2006;119(9):777-85. PMID: 16945613.
116. Baron JA, Beach M, Mandel JS, et al; Calcium Polyp Prevention Study Group. Calcium supplements for the prevention of colorectal adenomas. *N Engl J Med.* 1999;340(2):101-7. PMID: 9887161.
117. Jeon YJ, Myung SK, Lee EH, et al. Effects of beta-carotene supplements on cancer prevention: meta-analysis of randomized controlled trials. *Nutr Cancer.* 2011;63(8):1196-207. PMID: 21981610.
118. Fritz H, Kennedy D, Fergusson D, et al. Selenium and lung cancer: a systematic review and meta analysis. *PLoS One.* 2011;6(11):e26259. PMID: 22073154.
119. Flores-Mateo G, Navas-Acien A, Pastor-Barriuso R, et al. Selenium and coronary heart disease: a meta-analysis. *Am J Clin Nutr.* 2006;84(4):762-73. PMID: 17023702.
120. Wang L, Manson JE, Song Y, et al. Systematic review: vitamin D and calcium supplementation in prevention of cardiovascular events. *Ann Intern Med.* 2010;152(5):315-23. PMID: 20194238.
121. Autier P, Gandini S. Vitamin D supplementation and total mortality: a meta-analysis of randomized controlled trials. *Arch Intern Med.* 2007;167(16):1730-7. PMID: 17846391.
122. Bjelakovic G, Nikolova D, Simonetti RG, et al. Systematic review: primary and secondary prevention of gastrointestinal cancers with antioxidant supplements. *Aliment Pharmacol Ther.* 2008;28(6):689-703. PMID: 19145725.
123. Bjelakovic G, Nikolova D, Simonetti RG, et al. Antioxidant supplements for preventing gastrointestinal cancers. *Cochrane Database Syst Rev.* 2008;(3):CD004183. PMID: 18677777.
124. Bjelakovic G, Nikolova D, Gluud LL, et al. Antioxidant supplements for prevention of mortality in healthy participants and patients with various diseases. *Cochrane Database Syst Rev.* 2008(2):CD007176. PMID: 18425980.
125. Papaioannou D, Cooper KL, Carroll C, et al. Antioxidants in the chemoprevention of colorectal cancer and colorectal adenomas in the general population: a systematic review and meta-analysis. *Colorectal Dis.* 2011;13(10):1085-99. PMID: 20412095.

126. Chang YJ, Myung SK, Chung ST, et al. Effects of vitamin treatment or supplements with purported antioxidant properties on skin cancer prevention: a meta-analysis of randomized controlled trials. *Dermatology*. 2011;223(1):36-44. PMID: 21846961.
127. Rees K, Hartley L, Day C, et al. Selenium supplementation for the primary prevention of cardiovascular disease. *Cochrane Database Syst Rev*. 2013;(1):CD009671. PMID: 23440843.
128. Abner EL, Schmitt FA, Mendiondo MS, et al. Vitamin E and all-cause mortality: a meta-analysis. *Curr Aging Sci*. 2011;4(2):158-70. PMID: 21235492.
129. Alkhenizan A, Hafez K. The role of vitamin E in the prevention of cancer: a meta-analysis of randomized controlled trials. *Ann Saudi Med*. 2007;27(6):409-14. PMID: 18059122.
130. Shekelle P, Coulter I, Hardy M, et al. Effect of the Supplemental Use of Antioxidants Vitamin C, Vitamin E, and Coenzyme Q10 for the Prevention and Treatment of Cancer. AHRQ Publication No. 04-E003. Rockville, MD: Agency for Healthcare Research and Quality; 2003.
131. Shekelle PG, Morton SC, Jungvig LK, et al. Effect of supplemental vitamin E for the prevention and treatment of cardiovascular disease. *J Gen Intern Med*. 2004;19(4):380-9.
132. Bin Q, Hu X, Cao Y, et al. The role of vitamin E (tocopherol) supplementation in the prevention of stroke. A meta-analysis of 13 randomised controlled trials. *Thromb Haemost*. 2011;105(4):579-85. PMID: 21264448.
133. Mursu J, Robien K, Harnack LJ, et al. Dietary supplements and mortality rate in older women: the Iowa Women's Health Study. *Arch Intern Med*. 2011;171(18):1625-33. PMID: 21987192.
134. Tanvetyanon T, Bepler G. Beta-carotene in multivitamins and the possible risk of lung cancer among smokers versus former smokers: a meta-analysis and evaluation of national brands. *Cancer*. 2008;113(1):150-7. PMID: 18429004.
135. Cortes-Jofre M, Rueda JR, Corsini-Munoz G, et al. Drugs for preventing lung cancer in healthy people. *Cochrane Database Syst Rev*. 2012;(10):CD002141. PMID: 23076895.
136. Bolland MJ, Avenell A, Baron JA, et al. Effect of calcium supplements on risk of myocardial infarction and cardiovascular events: meta-analysis. *BMJ*. 2010;341:c3691. PMID: 20671013.
137. Bolland MJ, Grey A, Avenell A, et al. Calcium supplements with or without vitamin D and risk of cardiovascular events: reanalysis of the Women's Health Initiative limited access dataset and meta-analysis. *BMJ*. 2011;342:d2040. PMID: 21505219.
138. Prince RL, Devine A, Dhaliwal SS, et al. Effects of calcium supplementation on clinical fracture and bone structure: results of a 5-year, double-blind, placebo-controlled trial in elderly women. *Arch Intern Med*. 2006;166(8):869-75. PMID: 16636212.
139. Xiao Q, Murphy RA, Houston DK, et al. Dietary and supplemental calcium intake and cardiovascular disease mortality: the National Institutes of Health-AARP Diet and Health Study. *JAMA Intern Med*. 2013;173(8):639-46. PMID: 23381719.
140. Li K, Kaaks R, Linseisen J, et al. Associations of dietary calcium intake and calcium supplementation with myocardial infarction and stroke risk and overall cardiovascular mortality in the Heidelberg cohort of the European Prospective Investigation into Cancer and Nutrition study (EPIC-Heidelberg). *Heart*. 2012;98(12):920-5. PMID: 22626900.
141. Byers T. Anticancer vitamins du Jour—the ABCED's so far. *Am J Epidemiol*. 2010;172(1):1-3. PMID: 20562190.

142. Lichtenstein AH, Russell RM. Essential nutrients: food or supplements? Where should the emphasis be? *JAMA*. 2005;294(3):351-8. PMID: 16030280.
143. Klein EA, Thompson IM Jr, Tangen CM, et al. Vitamin E and the risk of prostate cancer: the Selenium and Vitamin E Cancer Prevention Trial (SELECT). *JAMA*. 2011;306(14):1549-56. PMID: 21990298.
144. Blot WJ, Li JY, Taylor PR, et al. Nutrition intervention trials in Linxian, China: supplementation with specific vitamin/mineral combinations, cancer incidence, and disease-specific mortality in the general population. *J Natl Cancer Inst*. 1993;85(18):1483-92. PMID: 8360931.
145. Lappe JM, Heaney RP. Why randomized controlled trials of calcium and vitamin D sometimes fail. *Dermatoendocrinol*. 2012;4(2):95-100. PMID: 22928064.
146. U.S. Preventive Services Task Force. Vitamin D and calcium supplementation to prevent fractures in adults: U.S. Preventive Services Task Force recommendation statement. *Ann Intern Med*. 2013;158(9):1-36. PMID: 23440177.
147. Marra MV, Boyar AP. Position of the American Dietetic Association: nutrient supplementation. *J Am Diet Assoc*. 2009;109(12):2073-85. PMID: 19957415.
148. American Heart Association. Vitamin and Mineral Supplements. Dallas: American Heart Association; 2013. Accessed at http://www.heart.org/HEARTORG/GettingHealthy/NutritionCenter/Vitamin-and-Mineral-Supplements_UCM_306033_Article.jsp on 7 October 2013.
149. American Institute for Cancer Research. Food, Nutrition, Physical Activity, and the Prevention of Cancer: A Global Perspective. Washington, DC: American Institute for Cancer Research; 2007.
150. National Institutes of Health State-of-the-Science Panel. National Institutes of Health State-of-the-Science Conference Statement: multivitamin/mineral supplements and chronic disease prevention. *Am J Clin Nutr*. 2007;85(1):257S-64S. PMID: 17209206.
151. Ezzedine K, Latreille J, Kesse-Guyot E, et al. Incidence of skin cancers during 5-year follow-up after stopping antioxidant vitamins and mineral supplementation. *Eur J Cancer*. 2010;46(18):3316-22. PMID: 20605091.
152. Hercberg S, Czernichow S, Galan P. Antioxidant vitamins and minerals in prevention of cancers: lessons from the SU.VI.MAX study. *Br J Nutr*. 2006;96(Suppl 1):S28-30. PMID: 16923246.
153. Hercberg S, Preziosi P, Briancon S, et al. A primary prevention trial using nutritional doses of antioxidant vitamins and minerals in cardiovascular diseases and cancers in a general population: the SU.VI.MAX study—design, methods, and participant characteristics. *Control Clin Trials*. 1998;19(4):336-51. PMID: 9683310.
154. Christen WG, Gaziano JM, Hennekens CH. Design of Physicians' Health Study II—a randomized trial of beta-carotene, vitamins E and C, and multivitamins, in prevention of cancer, cardiovascular disease, and eye disease, and review of results of completed trials. *Ann Epidemiol*. 2000;10(2):125-34. PMID: 10691066.
155. Albanes D, Heinonen OP, Huttunen JK, et al. Effects of alpha-tocopherol and beta-carotene supplements on cancer incidence in the Alpha-Tocopherol Beta-Carotene Cancer Prevention Study. *Am J Clin Nutr*. 1995;62(6 Suppl):1427S-30S. PMID: 7495243.

156. Albanes D, Heinonen OP, Taylor PR, et al. Alpha-tocopherol and beta-carotene supplements and lung cancer incidence in the Alpha-Tocopherol Beta-Carotene Cancer Prevention Study: effects of base-line characteristics and study compliance. *J Natl Cancer Inst*. 1996;88(21):1560-70. PMID: 8901854.
157. Heinonen OP, Huttenen JK, Albanes D. The Alpha-Tocopherol, Beta-Carotene Lung Cancer Prevention Study: design, methods, participant characteristics, and compliance. *Ann Epidemiol*. 1994;4(1):1-10. PMID: 8205268.
158. The Steering Committee of the Physicians'Health Study Research Group. Preliminary report: findings from the aspirin component of the ongoing Physicians' Health Study. *N Engl J Med*. 1988;318(4):262-4. PMID: 3275899.
159. Greenberg ER, Baron JA, Stevens MM, et al. The Skin Cancer Prevention Study: design of a clinical trial of beta-carotene among persons at high risk for nonmelanoma skin cancer. *Control Clin Trials*. 1989;10(2):153-66. PMID: 2666024.
160. Green A, Battistutta D, Hart V, et al. The Nambour Skin Cancer and Actinic Eye Disease Prevention Trial: design and baseline characteristics of participants. *Control Clin Trials*. 1994;15(6):512-22. PMID: 7851112.
161. Goodman GE, Omenn GS, Thornquist MD, et al. The Carotene and Retinol Efficacy Trial (CARET) to prevent lung cancer in high-risk populations: pilot study with cigarette smokers. *Cancer Epidemiol Biomarkers Prev*. 1993;2(4):389-96. PMID: 8348063.
162. Neuhouser ML, Barnett MJ, Kristal AR, et al. Dietary supplement use and prostate cancer risk in the Carotene and Retinol Efficacy Trial. *Cancer Epidemiol Biomarkers Prev*. 2009;18(8):2202-6. PMID: 19661078.
163. Omenn GS, Goodman GE, Thornquist MD, et al. The Carotene and Retinol Efficacy Trial (CARET) to prevent lung cancer in high-risk populations: pilot study with asbestos-exposed workers. *Cancer Epidemiol Biomarkers Prev*. 1993;2(4):381-7. PMID: 8348062.
164. Omenn GS, Goodman G, Thornquist M, et al. The Carotene and Retinol Efficacy Trial (CARET) for chemoprevention of lung cancer in high risk populations: smokers and asbestos-exposed workers. *Cancer Res*. 1994;54(7 Suppl):2038s-43s. PMID: 8137335.
165. Chae CU, Albert CM, Moorthy MV, et al. Vitamin E supplementation and the risk of heart failure in women. *Circ Heart Fail*. 2012;5(2):176-82. PMID: 22438520.
166. Dunn BK, Ryan A, Ford LG. Selenium and Vitamin E Cancer Prevention Trial: a nutrient approach to prostate cancer prevention. *Recent Results Cancer Res*. 2009;181:183-93. PMID: 19213568.
167. Dunn BK, Richmond ES, Minasian LM, et al. A nutrient approach to prostate cancer prevention: the Selenium and Vitamin E Cancer Prevention Trial (SELECT). *Nutr Cancer*. 2010;62(7):896-918. PMID: 20924966.
168. Klein EA, Thompson IM, Lippman SM, et al. SELECT: the Selenium and Vitamin E Cancer Prevention Trial: rationale and design. *Prostate Cancer Prostatic Dis*. 2000;3(3):145-51. PMID: 12497090.
169. Lippman SM, Goodman PJ, Klein EA, et al. Designing the Selenium and Vitamin E Cancer Prevention Trial (SELECT). *J Natl Cancer Inst*. 2005;97(2):94-102. PMID: 15657339.
170. Walsh PC. Re: Vitamin E and the risk of prostate cancer: the Selenium and Vitamin E Cancer Prevention Trial (SELECT). *J Urol*. 2012;187(5):1640-1. PMID: 22494720.

171. Wyatt G. Vitamin E increases prostate cancer risk in middle-aged men relative to placebo: no significant association observed with selenium, either alone or in combination with vitamin E. *Evid Based Nurs*. 2012;15(3):90-1. PMID: 22411161.
172. Reid ME, Duffield-Lillico AJ, Slate E, et al. The nutritional prevention of cancer: 400 mcg per day selenium treatment. *Nutr Cancer*. 2008;60(2):155-63. PMID: 18444146.
173. Stranges S, Marshall JR, Trevisan M, et al. Effects of selenium supplementation on cardiovascular disease incidence and mortality: secondary analyses in a randomized clinical trial. *Am J Epidemiol*. 2006;163(8):694-9. PMID: 16495471.
174. Moon TE, Levine N, Cartmel B, et al; Southwest Skin Cancer Prevention Study Group. Design and recruitment for retinoid Skin Cancer Prevention (SKICAP) trials. *Cancer Epidemiol Biomarkers Prev*. 1995;4(6):661-9. PMID: 8547834.
175. Lappe JM, Davies KM, Travers-Gustafson D, et al. Vitamin D status in a rural postmenopausal female population. *J Am Coll Nutr*. 2006 (5):395-402. PMID: 17031008.
176. Bolland MJ, Grey A, Gamble GD, et al. Risk of cardiovascular events with calcium/vitamin D: a reanalysis of the Women's Health Initiative. *J Bone Miner Res*. 2010;25:S50.
177. Brunner RL, Wactawski-Wende J, Caan BJ, et al. The effect of calcium plus vitamin D on risk for invasive cancer: results of the Women's Health Initiative (WHI) calcium plus vitamin D randomized clinical trial. *Nutr Cancer*. 2011;63(6):827-41. PMID: 21774589.
178. Chlebowski RT, Johnson KC, Kooperberg C, et al. Calcium plus vitamin D supplementation and the risk of breast cancer. *J Natl Cancer Inst*. 2008;100(22):1581-91. PMID: 19001601.
179. Ding EL, Mehta S, Fawzi WW, et al. Interaction of estrogen therapy with calcium and vitamin D supplementation on colorectal cancer risk: reanalysis of Women's Health Initiative randomized trial. *Int J Cancer*. 2008;122(8):1690-4. PMID: 18092326.
180. Hays J, Hunt JR, Hubbell FA, et al. The Women's Health Initiative recruitment methods and results. *Ann Epidemiol*. 2003;13(9 Suppl):S18-S77. PMID: 14575939.
181. Hsia J, Heiss G, Ren H, et al. Calcium/vitamin D supplementation and cardiovascular events. *Circulation*. 2007;115(7):846-54. PMID: 17309935.
182. Jackson RD, LaCroix AZ, Gass M, et al. Calcium plus vitamin D supplementation and the risk of fractures. *New Engl J Med*. 2006;354(7):669-83. PMID: 16481635.
183. LaCroix AZ, Kotchen J, Anderson G, et al. Calcium plus vitamin D supplementation and mortality in postmenopausal women: the Women's Health Initiative calcium-vitamin D randomized controlled trial. *J Gerontol A Biol Sci Med Sci*. 2009;64(5):559-67. PMID: 19221190.
184. Tang JY, Fu T, Leblanc E, et al. Calcium plus vitamin D supplementation and the risk of nonmelanoma and melanoma skin cancer: post hoc analyses of the Women's Health Initiative randomized controlled trial. *J Clin Oncol*. 2011;29(22):3078-84. PMID: 21709199.
185. Fu T, Tang JY, Leblanc E, et al. Calcium plus vitamin D supplementation and the risk of nonmelanoma and melanoma skin cancer. *J Invest Dermatol*. 2011;131(Suppl 1):S35.
186. Reid IR, Horne A, Mason B, et al. Effects of calcium supplementation on body weight and blood pressure in normal older women: a randomized controlled trial. *J Clin Endocrinol Metab*. 2005;90(7):3824-9. PMID: 15827103.

187. Harris RP, Helfand M, Woolf SH, et al. Current methods of the U.S. Preventive Services Task Force: a review of the process. *Am J Prev Med*. 2001;20(3 Suppl):21-35. PMID: 11306229.
188. Adjei AA. Calcitriol in Preventing Lung Cancer in Smokers and Former Smokers at High Risk of Lung Cancer. Buffalo, NY: Roswell Park Cancer Institute; 2012. Accessed at http://clinicaltrials.gov/ct2/show/NCT00690924 on 7 October 2013.
189. Camargo CA Jr. Effect of Vitamin D Supplementation on Cardiovascular and Respiratory Disease Event Rates, and the Incidence of Fractures. New Zealand: University of Auckland; 2011. Accessed at http://www.anzctr.org.au/trial_view.aspx?id=336777 on 7 October 2013.
190. Goossens ME, Buntinx F, Joniau S, et al. Designing the Selenium and Bladder Cancer Trial (SELEBLAT), a phase lll randomized chemoprevention study with selenium on recurrence of bladder cancer in Belgium. *BMC Urology*. 2012;12:8. PMID: 22436453.
191. Lance MP. Effect of Vitamin E and/or Selenium on Colorectal Polyps in Men Enrolled in SELECT Trial SWOG-S0000. Tucson, AZ: University of Arizona; 2011. Accessed at http://clinicaltrials.gov/ct2/show/NCT00706121 on 7 October 2013.
192. Lappe J. Clinical Trial of Vitamin D3 to Reduce Cancer Risk in Postmenopausal Women (CAPS). Fremont, Nebraska: Creighton University; 2012. Accessed at http://clinicaltrials.gov/show/NCT01052051 on 7 October 2013.
193. Lopez-Torres Hidalgo J; ANVITAD Group. Prevention of falls and fractures in old people by administration of calcium and vitamin D, randomized clinical trial. *BMC Public Health*. 2011;11:910. PMID: 22151975.
194. Manson JE, Bassuk SS, Lee IM, et al. The Vitamin D and Omega-3 Trial (VITAL): rationale and design of a large randomized controlled trial of vitamin D and marine omega-3 fatty acid supplements for the primary prevention of cancer and cardiovascular disease. *Contemp Clin Trials*. 2012;33(1):159-71. PMID: 21986389.
195. Peto J. Vitamin D and Longevity (VIDAL) Trial: Randomized Feasibility Study. London: London School of Hygiene and Tropical Medicine; 2012. Accessed at http://www.controlled-trials.com/ISRCTN46328341 on 7 October 2013.
196. Rhodes LE. The Effect of Green Tea and Vitamin C on Skin Health. Manchester: University of Manchester; 2009. Accessed at http://clinicaltrials.gov/ct2/show/NCT01032031 on 7 October 2013.
197. Tran B, Armstrong BK, Carlin JB, et al. Recruitment and results of a pilot trial of vitamin D supplementation in the general population of Australia. *J Clin Endocrinol Metab*. 2012;97(12):4473-80.
198. Tuomainen T, Virtanen J, Voutilainen S. Finnish Vitamin D Trial (FIND). Joensuu, Finland: University of Eastern Finland; 2011. Accessed at http://clinicaltrials.gov/ct2/show/NCT01463813 on 7 October 2013.

Figure 1. Analytic Framework

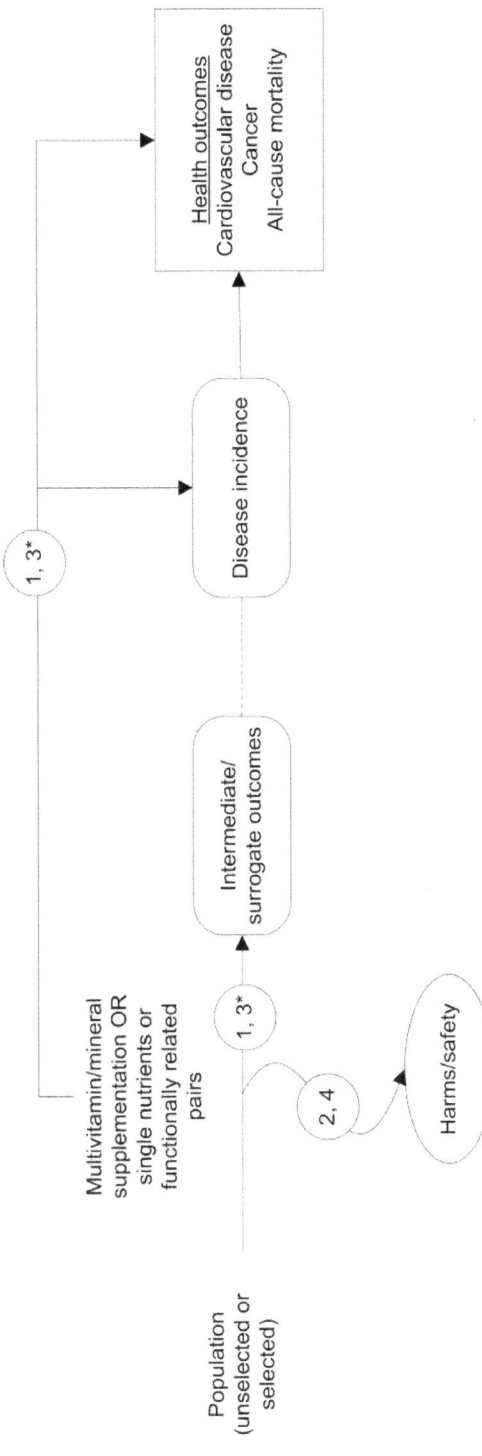

*Only includes intermediate outcomes (e.g., biomarkers) in trials reporting disease incidence.

Figure 2. Relative Risk for Any Cardiovascular Disease Incidence at Longest Followup Only, by Supplement

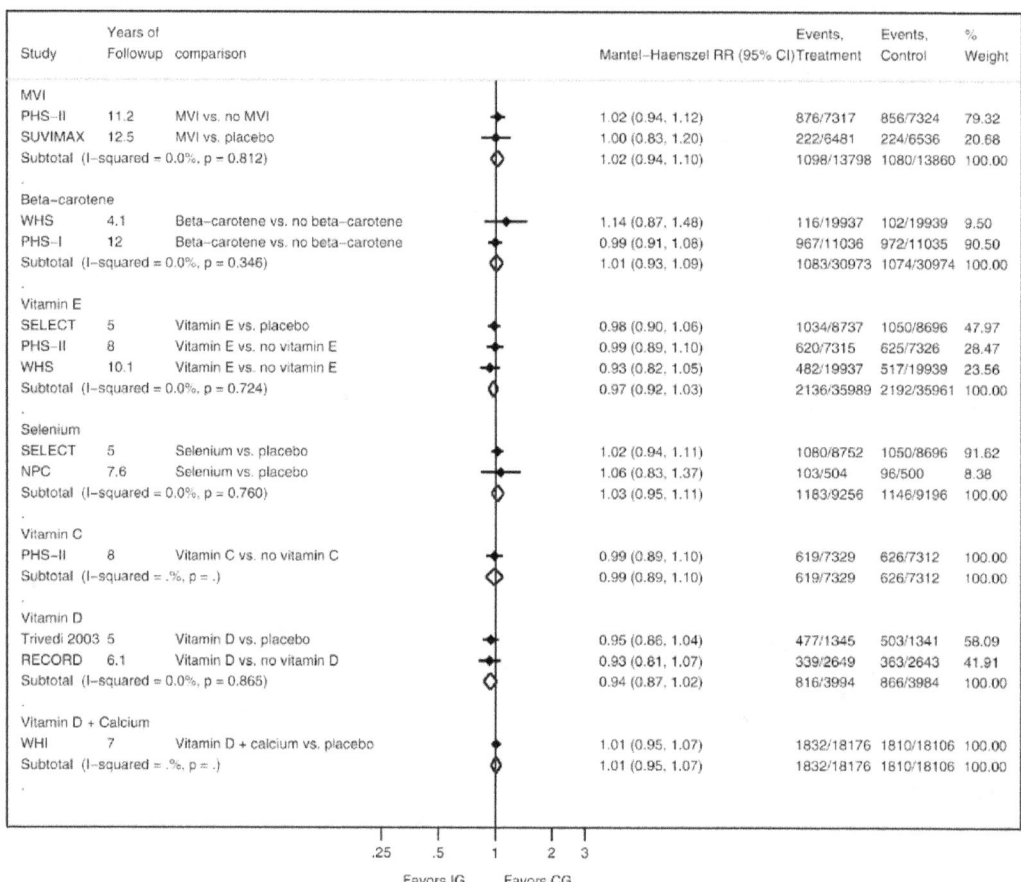

Abbreviations: CG = control group; CI = confidence interval; IG = intervention group; MVI = multivitamin; NPC = Nutritional Prevention of Cancer; PHS = Physician's Health Study; RECORD = Randomized Evaluation of Calcium or Vitamin D; RR = relative risk; SELECT = Selenium and Vitamin E Cancer Prevention Trial; SUVIMAX = Supplementation in VItamins and Mineral Antioxidants Study; WHI = Women's Health Initiative; WHS = Women's Health Study.

Figure 3. Relative Risk for Any Cancer Incidence at Longest Followup Only, by Supplement

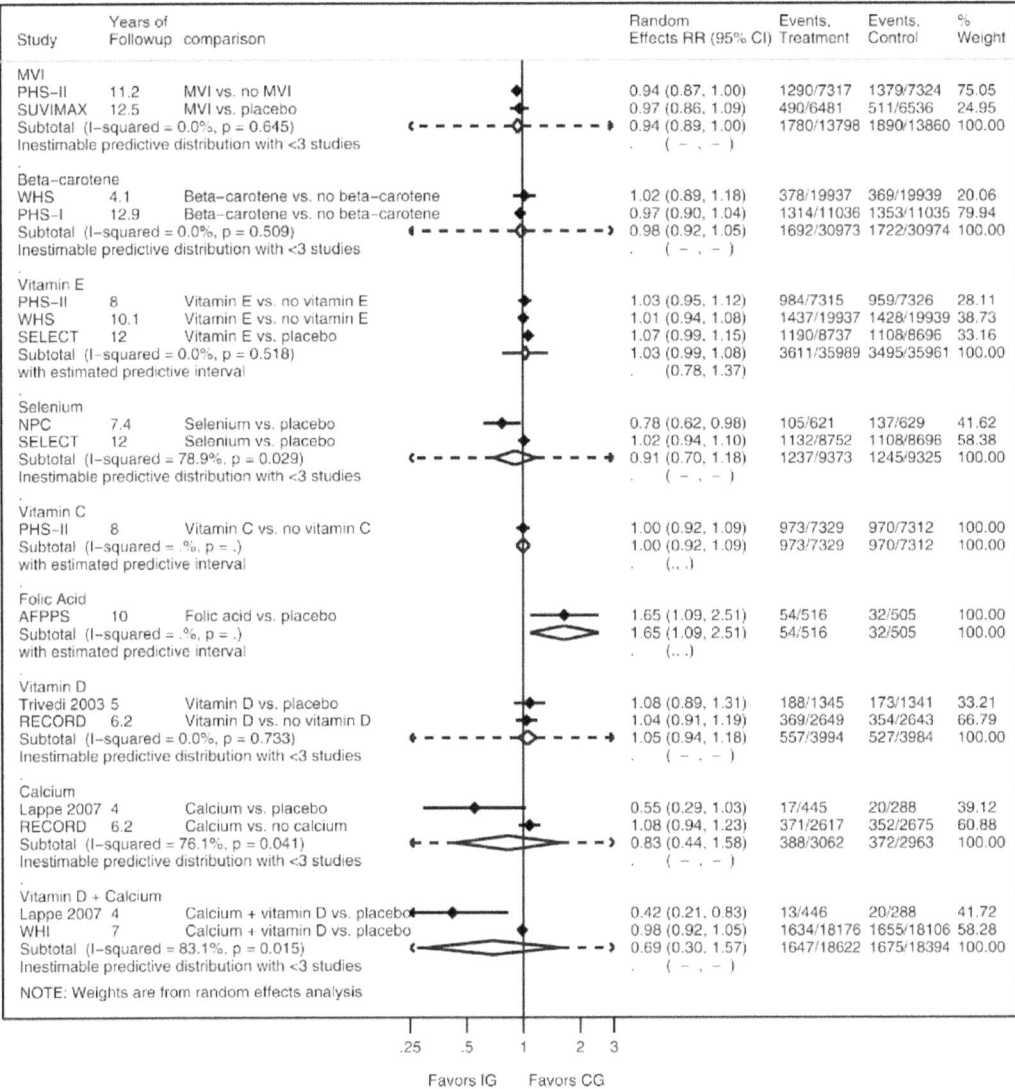

Abbreviations: AFPPS = Aspirin/Folate Polyp Prevention Study; CG = control group; CI = confidence interval; IG = intervention group; MVI = multivitamin; NPC = Nutritional Prevention of Cancer; PHS = Physician's Health Study; RECORD = Randomized Evaluation of Calcium or Vitamin D; RR = relative risk; SELECT = Selenium and Vitamin E Cancer Prevention Trial; SUVIMAX = Supplementation in VItamins and Mineral Antioxidants Study; WHI = Women's Health Initiative; WHS = Women's Health Study.

Figure 4. Relative Risk for All-Cause Mortality at Longest Followup Only, by Supplement

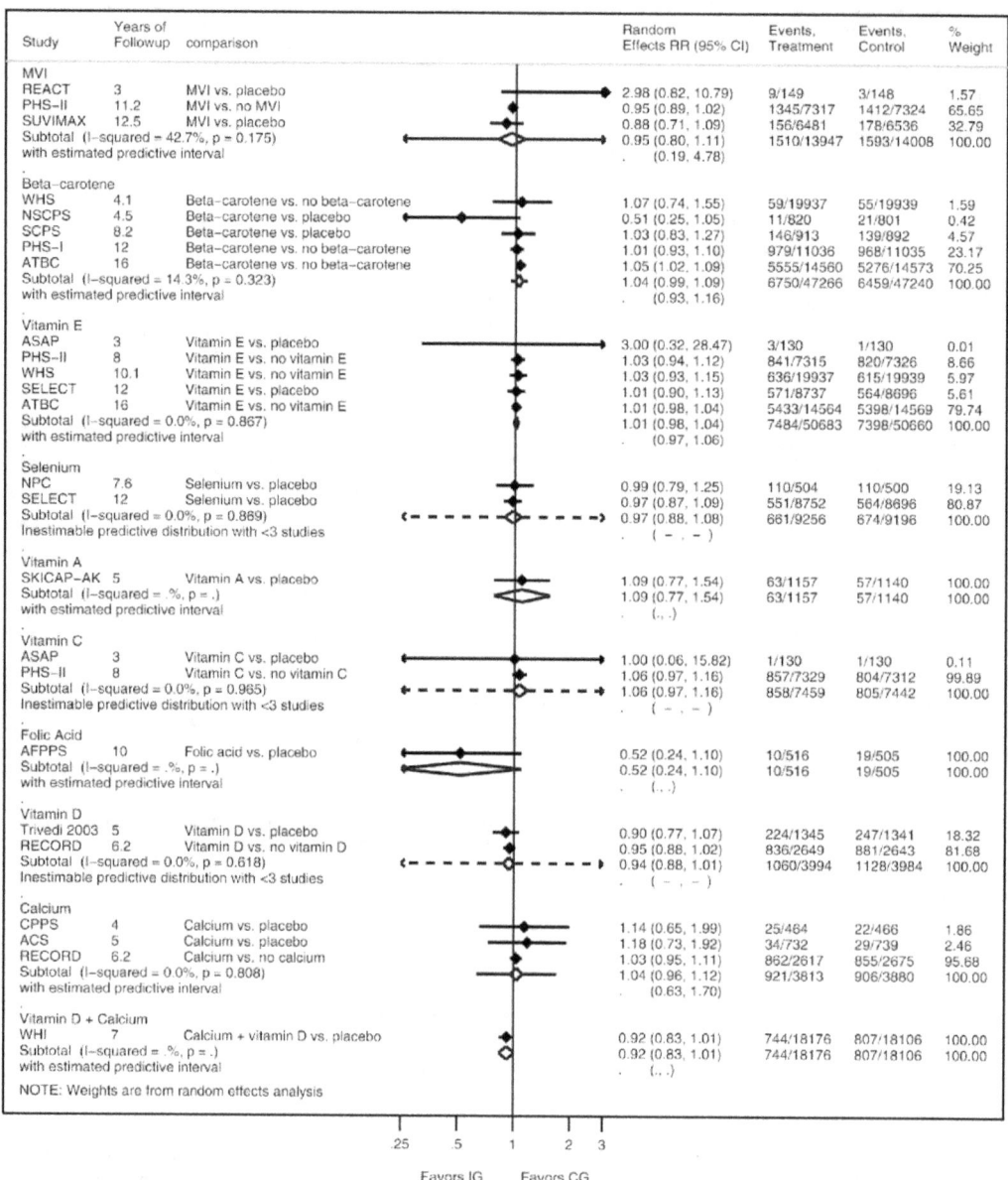

Abbreviations: AFPPS = Aspirin/Folate Polyp Prevention Study; ASAP = Antioxidant Supplementations in Atherosclerosis Prevention; ATBC = Alpha-Tocopherol Beta-Carotene Cancer Prevention; CG = control group; CI = confidence interval; IG = intervention group; MVI = multivitamin; NPC = Nutritional Prevention of Cancer; NSCPS = Nambour Skin Cancer Prevention Study; PHS = Physician's Health Study; REACT = Roche European American Cataract Trial; RECORD = Randomized Evaluation of Calcium or Vitamin D; RR = relative risk; SCPS = Skin Cancer Prevention Study; SELECT = Selenium and Vitamin E Cancer Prevention Trial; SKICAP-AK = Skin Cancer Prevention Trial-Actinic Keratoses; SUVIMAX = Supplementation in VItamins and Mineral Antioxidants Study; WHI = Women's Health Initiative; WHS = Women's Health Study.

Table 1. Dietary Reference Intake Definitions[2]

Term	Definition
Estimated Average Requirements	The average daily nutrient intake level that is estimated to meet the requirements of half of the healthy individuals in a particular life stage and sex group.
Recommended Dietary Allowance	The average daily dietary nutrient intake level that is sufficient to meet the nutrient requirements of nearly all (97% to 98%) healthy individuals in a particular life stage and sex group.
Adequate Intake	The recommended average daily intake level based on observed or experimentally determined approximations or estimates of nutrient intake by a group (or groups) of apparently healthy people that are assumed to be adequate; used when a Recommended Dietary Allowance cannot be determined.
Tolerable Upper Intake Level	The highest average daily nutrient intake level that is likely to pose no risk of adverse health effects to almost all individuals in the general population. As intake increases above the upper level, the potential risk of adverse effects may increase.

Table 2. Vitamin and Mineral Supplement Use in the United States, NHANES 2003–2006[10]

Supplement	Percent of U.S. population
Multivitamin	33
Vitamin B_6	29
Vitamin B_{12}	29
Vitamin C	31
Vitamin A	28
Vitamin E	29
Iron	18
Zinc	26
Magnesium	27
Selenium	19

Abbreviations: NHANES = National Health and Nutrition Examination Survey.

Table 3. Recommendations of Other Organizations

Organization and date of recommendation	Recommendation and rationale
American Dietetic Association, 2009[147]	The best nutrition-based strategy for promoting optimal health and reducing risk of chronic disease is to wisely choose a wide variety of foods. Additional nutrients from supplements can help some people meet their nutrition needs as specified by science-based nutrition standards, such as Dietary Reference Intake levels. Although multivitamin supplementation can be effective in helping meet recommended levels of some nutrients, evidence has not proven them to be effective in preventing chronic disease.
American Heart Association, 2013[148]	Recommends that healthy people get adequate nutrients by eating a variety of foods in moderation, rather than by taking supplements.
American Institute for Cancer Research, 2007[149]	Dietary supplements are not recommended for cancer prevention. High-dose supplements can be protective or cause cancer; however, such studies are not applicable to widespread use (i.e., the general population), in which the balance of benefits and harms (e.g., unexpected side effects) cannot be confidently predicted. The American Institute for Cancer Research suggests increasing nutrients through diet.
National Institutes of Health, 2007[150]	The present evidence is insufficient to recommend either for or against the use of multivitamins (any supplement containing three or more vitamins and minerals but no herbs, hormones, or drugs; each at a dose less than the tolerable upper intake level determined by the U.S. Food and Nutrition Board) to prevent chronic disease.

Table 4. Framingham Heart Study Average Annual Incidence Rates* of Cardiovascular Disease in the United States, 1980–2003[17]

Condition	Age group (years)	Men	Women
Cardiovascular disease**	45–54	10.1	4.2
	55–64	21.4	8.9
	65–74	34.6	20.0
	75–84	29.2	40.2
	85–94	74.4	65.2
Myocardial infarction	45–54	4.6	0.8
	55–64	11.4	3.2
	65–74	11.9	5.7
	75–84	22.8	11.0
	85–94	24.5	17.3
Stroke	45–54	1.3	1.4
	55–64	4.3	2.2
	65–74	11.1	7.0
	75–84	19.6	17.1
	85–94	16.2	27.1
Heart failure	45–54	1.5	0.8
	55–64	3.3	1.3
	65–74	9.2	4.6
	75–84	22.3	14.8
	85–94	43.0	30.6
Angina pectoris	45–54	4.8	1.1
	55–64	8.9	4.0
	65–74	9.9	5.6
	75–84	13.0	6.2
	85–94	7.4	3.2

*Per 1,000 person-years.
*Coronary heart disease, heart failure, cerebrovascular accident, or intermittent claudication.

Table 5. Centers for Disease Control and Prevention Age-Adjusted Mortality Rates* of Cardiovascular Disease in the United States Based on I00-I99 Codes, 2009[17]

Race/ethnicity	Men	Women
White	281.4	190.4
Black	387.0	267.9
Asian/Pacific Islander	171.6	118.1
American Indian/Alaskan Native	196.5	129.4
Hispanic	198.9	138.6

*Per 1,000 individuals.

Table 6. SEER Incidence Rates* of Cancer in the United States, 2005–2009

Cancer site	Race/ethnicity	Men	Women
Any	White	542.7	423.1
	Black	627.1	398.3
	Asian/Pacific Islander	342.6	299.4
	American Indian/Alaskan Native	352.7	313.8
	Hispanic	402.0	324.1
Prostate	White	146.9	
	Black	236.0	
	Asian/Pacific Islander	85.4	
	American Indian/Alaskan Native	78.4	
	Hispanic	125.9	
Breast	White		127.3
	Black		121.2
	Asian/Pacific Islander		94.5
	American Indian/Alaskan Native		80.6
	Hispanic		92.7
Colorectal	White	53.1	39.2
	Black	66.9	50.3
	Asian/Pacific Islander	44.9	34.2
	American Indian/Alaskan Native	45.2	38.0
	Hispanic	45.2	31.5
Lung	White	76.4	55.1
	Black	99.9	52.6
	Asian/Pacific Islander	52.2	28.8
	American Indian/Alaskan Native	51.9	37.4
	Hispanic	40.5	25.8

*Per 1,000 individuals.

Abbreviation: SEER = Surveillance Epidemiology and End Results.

Table 7. SEER Mortality Rates* of Cancer in the United States, 2005–2009

Cancer site	Race/ethnicity	Men	Women
Any	White	216.7	150.8
	Black	288.3	174.6
	Asian/Pacific Islander	132.6	93.2
	American Indian/Alaskan Native	184.9	135.9
	Hispanic	146.3	100.5
Prostate	White	21.7	
	Black	53.1	
	Asian/Pacific Islander	10.0	
	American Indian/Alaskan Native	19.7	
	Hispanic	17.8	
Breast	White		22.4
	Black		31.6
	Asian/Pacific Islander		11.9
	American Indian/Alaskan Native		16.6
	Hispanic		14.9
Colorectal	White	19.5	13.6
	Black	29.8	19.8
	Asian/Pacific Islander	13.1	9.6
	American Indian/Alaskan Native	18.8	14.6
	Hispanic	15.3	10.2
Lung	White	65.3	40.8
	Black	82.6	38.0
	Asian/Pacific Islander	35.9	18.5
	American Indian/Alaskan Native	48.3	33.2
	Hispanic	30.8	14.0

*Average age-adjusted annual rates per 100,000 individuals.

Abbreviation: SEER = Surveillance Epidemiology and End Results.

Table 8. Multivitamin Evidence Summary

Study Quality	Study design Followup (max)	Supplement* and treatment duration	N	Mean age (y)	% Female	CVD incidence	Cancer incidence	Mortality	Harms	Comments
SU.VI.MAX[49,54-56,58,151-153] Good	RCT 13 years	Multivitamin 7.5 years (median)	13,017	49	59	Any: ↔ MI: NR Stroke: NR	Any: ↔ Lung: ↔ CRC: ↔ Prostate: ↔ Breast: ↔ Other: ↔	↔	↔	Protective effect against cancer in men (↓) but not women (↔)‡
PHS-II[50,57,154] Good	2x2x2x2 factorial RCT 11.2 years	Multivitamin 11.2 years (median)	14,641	64	0	Any: ↔ MI: ↔† Stroke: ↔	Any: ↓ Lung: ↔ CRC: ↔ Prostate: ↔ Breast: NA Other: ↔	↔	↔	Minor side effects (↔), rashes (↑), and bleeding (↑)
REACT[51] Good	RCT 3 years	Multivitamin 3 years	297	66	59	NA	NA	↔	↔	
Graat 2002[52] Good	2x2 RCT 1.3 years	Multivitamin (alone or in combination with vitamin E 200 mg) 1.3 years	652	73	50	NA	NA	NA	↔	Acute respiratory infections (↔)
NHS[53] Good	Prospective cohort 18 years	Multivitamin NR	72,337	58	100	NA	NA	NA	↑	Hip fractures among current and former multivitamin users (↑)

*See Table 10 for vitamin and mineral components and their dosages for each study.
†Decreased risk for fatal myocardial infarction (p=0.048).
‡Statistically significant protective effect for any cancer in men but not women.

Abbreviations: CRC = colorectal cancer; CVD = cardiovascular disease; MI = myocardial infarction; NA = not applicable; NHS = Nurses' Health Study; NR = not reported; PHS-II = Physician's Health Study II; RCT = randomized, controlled trial; REACT = Roche European American Cataract Trial; SU.VI.MAX = Supplementation in VItamins and Mineral AntioXidants Study; y = years.

Legend: ↑ (statistically significant increase in risk of outcome from supplementation), ↔ (no statistically significant difference between intervention groups), ↓ (statistically significant decrease in risk of outcome from supplementation).

Table 9. Vitamin and Mineral Components of the Multivitamin Studies

Vitamin/mineral	SU.VI.MAX[49]	PHS-II[50]	REACT[51]	Graat[52]	NHS[53]
Not described					X
Beta-carotene	6 mg	*	6 mg	1.2 mg	
Biotin		30 mcg		150 mcg	
Boron		150 mcg			
Calcium		200 mg		74 mg	
Chloride		72.6 mg			
Chromium		130 mcg		25 mcg	
Copper		2 mg		1.0 mg	
Folic acid		400 mcg		200 mcg	
Iodine		150 mcg		100 mcg	
Iron		4 mg		4.0 mg	
Magnesium		100 mg		30 mg	
Manganese		3.5 mg		1.0 mg	
Molybdenum		160 mcg		25 mcg	
Niacin		20 mg			
Nickel		5 mcg			
Pantothenic acid		10 mg			
Phosphorus		48 mg		49 mg	
Potassium		80 mcg			
Riboflavin		1.7 mg			
Selenium	100 mcg	20 mcg		25 mcg	
Silicon		2 mg		2 mcg	
Thiamin		1.5 mg			
Vanadium		10 mcg			
Vitamin A		5,000 IU		600 mg	
Vitamin B_1				1.4 mg	
Vitamin B_{12}		25 mcg		1 mcg	
Vitamin B_2				1.6 mg	
Vitamin B_3				18 mg	
Vitamin B_5				6 mg	
Vitamin B_6		3 mg		2.0 mg	
Vitamin C	120 mg	60 mg	250 mg	60 mg	
Vitamin D		400 IU		5 mcg	
Vitamin E	30 mg	45 IU	200 mg	10 mg	
Vitamin K		10 mcg		30 mcg	
Zinc	20 mg	15 mg		10 mg	

*40% was supplemented with vitamin A.

Table 10. Cardiovascular Disease Incidence and Mortality Among Multivitamin Studies

Outcome	Study	Comparison	Mean followup (y)	Intervention, # of subjects with event (%)	Comparator, # of subjects with event (%)	RR or HR	95% CI	P-value
Ischemic CVD incidence*	SU.VI.MAX[49,56]	MVI vs. placebo	7.5	134/6,481 (2.1)	137/6,536 (2.1)	0.97†	0.77 to 1.20	0.80
Any CVD incidence‖	PHS-II[57]	MVI vs. no MVI	12.5	222/6,481 (3)	224/6,539 (4)	0.97†	0.80 to 1.17	0.73
	PHS-II[57]	MVI vs. no MVI	11.2	876/7,317 (12)	856/7,324 (11.7)	1.01‡	0.91 to 1.10	0.91
MI incidence	PHS-II[57]	MVI vs. no MVI	11.2	317/7,317 (4.3)	335/7,324 (4.6)	0.93‡	0.80 to 1.09	0.39
Stroke incidence	PHS-II[57]§	MVI vs. no MVI	11.2	332/7,317 (4.5)	311/7,324 (4.2)	1.06‡	0.91 to 1.23	0.48
Any CVD death	PHS-II[57]	MVI vs. no MVI	11.2	408/7,317 (5.6)	421/7,324 (5.7)	0.95‡	0.83 to 1.09	0.47
Fatal MI	PHS-II[57]	MVI vs. no MVI	11.2	27/7,317 (0.4)	43/7,324 (0.6)	0.61‡	0.38 to 0.995	0.048
Fatal stroke	PHS-II[57]	MVI vs. no MVI	11.2	89/7,317 (1.2)	76/7,324 (1.0)	1.16‡	0.85 to 1.58	0.34

*Includes fatal and nonfatal ischemic CVD events.
†RR adjusted by age and sex unless otherwise noted.
‡HR adjusted by age, study cohort, beta-carotene assignment, and vitamin E and C assignment and stratified by CVD at baseline.
§Ischemic and hemorrhagic stroke reported separately, no significant difference between groups for either outcome.
‖Includes nonfatal MI, nonfatal stroke, and CVD death.

Abbreviations: CI = confidence interval; CVD = cardiovascular disease; HR = hazard ratio; MI = myocardial infarction; MVI = multivitamin; PHS-II = Physician's Health Study II; RR = relative risk; SU.VI.MAX = Supplementation in Vitamins and Mineral Antioxidants Study; y = years.

Table 11. Cancer Incidence and Mortality Among Multivitamin Studies

Outcome	Study	Comparison	Mean followup (y)	Intervention, # of subjects with event (%)	Comparator, # of subjects with event (%)	RR or HR	95% CI	P-value
All cancer sites incidence	SU.VI.MAX[49,55,56]	MVI vs. placebo	7.5	267/6,481 (4.1)	295/6,536 (4.5)	0.90†	0.76 to 1.06	0.19
	PHS-II[50]	MVI vs. no MVI	12.5	490/6,481 (7.5)	511/6,536 (7.8)	0.93†	0.82 to 1.05	NSD
	PHS-II[50]	MVI vs. no MVI	11.2	1,290/7,317 (17.6)	1,379/7,324 (18.8)	0.92*	0.86 to 0.998	0.04
Breast cancer incidence	SU.VI.MAX[49,55,56]	MVI vs. placebo	7.5	95/3,859 (2.5)	100/3,820 (2.6)	NR	NR	NR
Prostate cancer incidence	SU.VI.MAX[49,55,56]	MVI vs. placebo	8.9	49/2,569 (1.9)	54/2,572 (2.1)	0.88‡	0.60 to 1.29	NSD
	PHS-II[50]	MVI vs. no MVI	11.2	683/6,988 (9.8)	690/6,992 (9.9)	0.98*	0.88 to 1.09	0.76
Colorectal cancer incidence	PHS-II[50]	MVI vs. no MVI	11.2	99/7,255 (1.4)	111/7,264 (1.5)	0.89*	0.68 to 1.17	0.39
Lung cancer incidence	PHS-II[50]	MVI vs. no MVI	11.2	74/7,300 (1.0)	88/7,310 (1.2)	0.84*	0.61 to 1.25	0.26
Any cancer death	PHS-II[50]	MVI vs. no MVI	11.2	403/7,317 (5.5)	456/7,324 (6.2)	0.88*	0.77 to 1.01	0.07
Prostate cancer death	PHS-II[50]	MVI vs. no MVI	11.2	707/7,317 (1.0)	78/7,324 (1.1)	0.91*	0.66 to 1.26	0.58
Colorectal cancer death	PHS-II[50]	MVI vs. no MVI	11.2	37/7,317 (0.5)	39/7,324 (0.5)	0.95*	0.60 to 1.48	0.81
Lung cancer death	PHS-II[50]	MVI vs. no MVI	11.2	65/7,317 (0.9)	73/7,324 (1.0)	0.89*	0.64 to 1.25	0.50

*HR adjusted by age, study cohort, and randomized treatment assignment; stratified by baseline cancer.
†RR adjusted by age and sex unless otherwise noted.
‡HR, adjustment not reported.

Abbreviations: CI = confidence interval; HR = hazard ratio; MVI = multivitamin; NR = not reported; NSD = no significant difference; PHS-II = Physician's Health Study II; RR = relative risk; SU.VI.MAX = Supplementation in Vitamins and Mineral Antioxidants Study; y = years.

Table 12. All-Cause Mortality Among Multivitamin Studies

Study	Comparison	Mean followup (y)	Intervention, # of deaths (%)	Comparator, # of deaths (%)	RR or HR	95% CI	P-value
SU.VI.MAX[49,56]	MVI vs. placebo	7.5	76/6,481 (1.2)	98/6,536 (1.5)	0.77*	0.57 to 1.00	0.09
		12.5	156/6,481 (2.4)	178/6,536 (2.7)	0.87*	0.70 to 1.04	0.19
PHS-II[50]	MVI vs. no MVI	11.2	1,345/7,317 (18.4)	1,412/7,324 (19.3)	0.94†	0.88 to 1.02	0.13
REACT[51]	MVI vs. placebo	3	9/149 (6)	3/148 (2)	NR	NR	0.07

*Adjusted by age and sex unless otherwise noted.
†HR adjusted for age, study cohort, and randomized assignment (beta-carotene, vitamin E, and vitamin C) and stratified by baseline cardiovascular disease and cancer.

Abbreviations: CI = confidence interval; HR = hazard ratio; MVI = multivitamin; NR = not reported; PHS-II = Physician's Health Study II; REACT = Roche European American Cataract Trial; RR = relative risk; SU.VI.MAX = Supplementation in VItamins and Mineral AntioXidants Study; y = years.

Table 13. Beta-Carotene Evidence Summary

Study Quality	Study design Followup	Supplement and dose Supplement duration	N	Mean age (y)	% Female	CVD incidence	Cancer incidence	Mortality	Harms	Comments
ATBC[59,66,69-73,76-78,87,88,155-157] Good	2x2 factorial RCT 16 years (max)	Beta-carotene 20 mg qd (alone or in combination with vitamin E 50 mg qd) 6.1 years (mean) (range, 5 to 8 years)	29,133	57	0	NR	Any: ↔ Lung: ↑* CRC: ↔† Prostate Breast: NA Other: ↔	↑	↓	Baseline population at high risk for lung cancer (all smokers)
PHS-I[61,65,68,158] Good	2x2 factorial RCT 12 years	Beta-carotene 50 mg qod (alone or in combination with aspirin) 12 years (mean)	22,071	NR	0	Any: ↔ MI: ↔ Stroke: ↔	Any: ↔ Lung: ↔ CRC: ↔ Prostate: ↔ Breast: NA Other: ↑‡	↔	↔	
WHS[62] Good	2x2x2 RCT 4.1 years	Beta-carotene 50 mg qod (alone or in combination with vitamin E 600 IU qod and/or aspirin) 2.1 years (median) (range, 0 to 2.72 years)	39,876	55	100	Any: ↔ MI: ↔ Stroke: ↔	Any: ↔ Lung: ↔ CRC: ↔ Prostate: NA Breast: ↔ Other: ↔	↔	↔	
SCPS[63,75,159] Good	RCT 8.2 years	Beta-carotene 50 mg qd 5 years	1,805	63	31	NA	NA	↔	↔	
NSCPS[64,160] Good	2x2 factorial RCT 4.5 years	Beta-carotene 30 mg qd (alone or in combination with topical sunscreen) 4.5 years	1,621	49	56	NA	NA	↔	↔	
CARET[60,67,74,161-164] Good	RCT 11 years	Beta-carotene 30 mg qd and vitamin A 25,000 IU qd NR	18,314	58	34	NA	Any: ↔ Lung: ↑* CRC: ↔ Prostate: ↔ Breast: ↔ Other: ↔	↑	↔	Baseline population at high risk for lung cancer (smokers or asbestos-exposed workers)

*Including deaths due to lung cancer.

Table 13. Beta-Carotene Evidence Summary

†Late negative effect after 14 years of followup.
‡Increased risk for thyroid and bladder cancer after 12 years of followup.

Abbreviations: ATBC = Alpha-Tocopherol Beta-Carotene Cancer Prevention; bid = twice daily; CARET = Carotene and Retinol Efficacy Trial; CRC = colorectal cancer; CVD = cardiovascular disease; MI = myocardial infarction; NA = not applicable; NR = not reported; NSCPS = Nambour Skin Cancer Prevention Study; PHS-I = Physician's Health Study I; qd = once daily; qod = every other day; RCT = randomized, controlled trial; SCPS = Skin Cancer Prevention Study; WHS = Women's Health Study; y = years.

Legend: ↑ (statistically significant increase in risk of outcome from supplementation), ↔ (no statistically significant difference between intervention groups), ↓ (statistically significant decrease in risk of outcome from supplementation).

Table 14. Cardiovascular Disease Incidence and Mortality Among Beta-Carotene Studies

Outcome	Study	Comparison	Mean followup (y)	Intervention, # of subjects with events (%)	Comparator, # of subjects with events (%)	RR*	95% CI	P-value
Any CVD§	PHS-I[61]	Beta-carotene vs. no beta-carotene	12	967/11,036 (8.8)	972/11,035 (8.8)	1.0	0.91 to 1.09	0.09
	WHS[62]	Beta-carotene vs. no beta-carotene	4.1	116/19,937 (0.6)	102/19,939 (0.5)	1.14	0.87 to 1.49	0.34
MI incidence	PHS-I[61]	Beta-carotene vs. no beta-carotene	12	468/11,036 (4.2)	489/11,035 (4.4)	0.96	0.84 to 1.09	0.50
	WHS[62]	Beta-carotene vs. no beta-carotene	4.1	42/19,937 (0.2)	50/19,939 (0.3)	0.84	0.56 to 1.27	0.41
Stroke incidence	PHS-I[61]	Beta-carotene vs. no beta-carotene	12	367/11,036 (3.3)	382/11,035 (3.5)	0.96	0.83 to 1.11	0.60
	WHS[62]	Beta-carotene vs. no beta-carotene	4.1	61/19,937 (0.3)	43/19,939 (0.2)	1.42	0.96 to 2.10	0.08
Any CVD death	NSCPS[64]	Beta-carotene vs. placebo	4.5	6/820 (0.7)	12/801 (1.5)	NR	NR	NR
	SCPS[75]	Beta-carotene vs. placebo	8.2	68/913 (7.4)	59/892 (6.6)	1.16	0.82 to 1.64	0.41
	WHS[62]	Beta-carotene vs. no beta-carotene	4.1	14/19,937 (0.1)	12/19,939 (0.1)	1.17	0.54 to 2.53	0.69
	PHS-I[61]	Beta-carotene vs. no beta-carotene	12	338/11,036 (3.1)	313/11,035 (2.8)	1.09	0.93 to 1.27	0.28
	CARET[67,74]	Beta-carotene + vitamin A vs. placebo	4	NR	NR	1.26	0.99 to 1.61	NR
			6†	354/8,744 (4)	319/8,396 (3.8)	1.02	0.88 to 1.19	NR

*Adjusted for age (PHS-I, WHS), random assignment (PHS-I, WHS), and/or multivariate (SCPS: age, sex, study center, previous skin cancer, age at diagnosis, skin type, smoking status, baseline plasma levels); unadjusted (CARET).
†Not cumulative, total number of deaths during 6-year posttrial period only (i.e., does not include deaths during supplementation phase).
§Includes nonfatal strokes, nonfatal MI, and cardiovascular-related death.

Abbreviations: CARET = Carotene and Retinol Efficacy Trial; CI = confidence interval; CVD = cardiovascular disease; MI = myocardial infarction; NSCPS = Nambour Skin Cancer Prevention Study; NR = not reported; PHS-I = Physician's Health Study I; RR = relative risk; SCPS = Skin Cancer Prevention Study; WHS = Women's Health Study; y = years.

Table 15. Cancer Incidence and Mortality Among Beta-Carotene Studies

Outcome	Study	Comparison	Mean followup (y)	Intervention, # of subjects with events (%)	Comparator, # of subjects with events (%)	RR	95% CI	P-value
Any cancer incidence	PHS-I[61,68]	Beta-carotene vs. no beta-carotene	12	1,273/11,036 (11.5)	1,293/11,035 (11.7)	0.98	0.91 to 1.06	0.65
			12.9	1,314/11,036 (11.9)	1,353/11,035 (12.3)	1.0	0.9 to 1.0	0.41
	WHS[62]	Beta-carotene vs. no beta-carotene	4.1	378/19,937 (1.9)	369/19,939 (1.9)	1.03	0.89 to 7.18	0.73
Lung cancer incidence	ATBC*[59,73]	Beta-carotene vs. no beta-carotene	6.1	474/14,560 (3.3)	402/14,573 (2.8)	1.18	1.03 to 1.36	0.01
			8	481/14,560 (3.3)	414/14,573 (2.8)	1.17	1.02 to 1.33	NR
			11¶	266/12,559 (2.1)	232/12,724 (1.8)	1.17	0.98 to 1.39	NR
			14¶	262/11,276 (2.3)	277/11,562 (2.4)	0.97	0.82 to 1.15	NR
	PHS-I[61,68]	Beta-carotene vs. no beta-carotene	12	82/11,036 (0.7)	88/11,035 (0.8)	0.93	0.69 to 1.26	NR
			12.9	85/11,036 (0.8)	93/11,035 (0.8)	0.90	0.7 to 1.2	0.54
	WHS[62]	Beta-carotene vs. no beta-carotene	4.1	31/19,937 (0.2)	21/19,939 (0.1)	NR	NR	NR
	CARET[60,57,74]	Beta-carotene + vitamin A vs. placebo	4	229/9,420 (2.4)	159/8,894 (1.8)	1.28	1.04 to 1.57	0.02
			6	376/8,744 (4.3)	311/8,396 (3.7)	1.12	0.97 to 1.31	0.13
Breast cancer incidence	WHS[62]	Beta-carotene vs. no beta-carotene	4.1	169/19,937 (0.8)	168/19,939 (0.8)	NR	NR	NR
	CARET[60,57,74]	Beta-carotene + vitamin A vs. placebo	4	59/3,208 (1.8)	65/3,081 (2.1)	0.78	0.55 to 1.12	0.18
Prostate cancer incidence	ATBC*[59,73,157]	Beta-carotene vs. no beta-carotene	6.1†	136/14,560 (0.9)	110/14,573 (0.8)	1.23	0.96 to 1.59	0.088
			8	138/14,560 (0.9)	110/14,573 (0.8)	1.26	0.98 to 162	NR
			11¶	149/12,614 (1.2)	128/12,776 (1)	1.18	0.94 to 1.50	NR
			14¶	193/11,237 (1.7)	202/11,533 (1.8)	0.98	0.81 to 1.20	NR
	PHS-I[61,68]	Beta-carotene vs. no beta-carotene	12	520/11,036 (4.7)	527/11,035 (4.8)	0.98	0.88 to 1.11	NR
			12.9	551/11,036 (5)	566/11,035 (5.1)	1.0	0.9 to 1.1	0.62
	CARET[60,57,74]	Beta-carotene + vitamin A vs. placebo	4	161/6,212 (2.6)	139/5,813 (2.4)	1.01	0.80 to 1.27	0.95
			11	462/6,197 (7.4)	428/5,803 (7.4)	NR	NR	NSD
Colorectal cancer incidence	ATBC*[59,73,157]	Beta-carotene vs. no beta-carotene	6.1†	69/14,560 (0.5)	66/14,573 (0.5)	1.05	0.75 to 1.47	NR
			8	69/14,560 (0.5)	66/14,573 (0.5)	1.05	0.75 to 1.47	NR
			11¶	47/12,670 (0.4)	45/12,819 (0.4)	1.06	0.70 to 160	NR
			14¶	73/11,373 (0.6)	40/11,631 (0.3)	1.88	1.28 to 2.76	NR
	PHS-I[61,68]	Beta-carotene vs. no beta-carotene	12	167/11,036 (1.5)	174/11,035 (1.6)	0.96	0.78 to 1.18	NR
			12.9	170/11,036 (1.5)	176/11,035 (1.6)	0.97	0.78 to 1.19	NR
	WHS[62]‡	Beta-carotene vs. no beta-carotene	4.1	34/19,937 (0.2)	34/19,939 (0.2)	1.0	0.8 to 1.2	NR
	CARET[60,57,74]	Beta-carotene + vitamin A vs. placebo	4	56/9,420 (0.6)	50/8,894 (0.6)	1.02	0.70 to 1.50	0.91
Any cancer death	NSCPS[54]	Beta-carotene vs. placebo	4.5	3/820 (0.4)	7/801 (0.9)	NR	NR	NR
	SCPS[75]	Beta-carotene vs. placebo	8.2	38/913 (4.2)	44/892 (4.9)	0.83	0.54 to 1.29	0.41
	WHS[62]	Beta-carotene vs. no beta-carotene	4.1	31/19,937 (0.2)	28/19,939 (0.1)	1.11	0.67 to 1.85	0.69
	PHS-I[61]	Beta-carotene vs. no beta-carotene	12	386/11,036 (3.5)	380/11,035 (3.4)	1.02	0.89 to 1.18	0.76

Table 15. Cancer Incidence and Mortality Among Beta-Carotene Studies

Outcome	Study	Comparison	Mean followup (y)	Intervention, # of subjects with events (%)	Comparator, # of subjects with events (%)	RR	95% CI	P-value
Lung cancer death	SCPS[75]	Beta-carotene vs. placebo	8.2	13/913 (1.4)	17/892 (1.9)	NR	NR	NR
	PHS-I[61]	Beta-carotene vs. no beta-carotene	12	63/11,036 (0.6)	62/11,035 (0.6)	NR	NR	NR
	ATBC[59,73]	Beta-carotene vs. no beta-carotene	6.1	302/14,560 (2.1)	262/14,573 (1.8)	NR	NR	0.08
			12.1	1,524/5,298§ (28.8)		NR	NR	
	CARET[60,67,74]	Beta-carotene + vitamin A vs. placebo	4	NR	NR	1.17	1.03 to 1.33	0.02
			6§	1,225/8,744 (14)	1,047/8,396 (12.5)	1.08	0.99 to 1.17	0.07
Prostate cancer death	ATBC[76]	Beta-carotene vs. no beta-carotene	6	33/14,560 (0.2)	29/14,573 (0.2)	1.15	0.70 to 1.89	NR

*Overall 6-year posttrial followup: lung cancer RR, 1.06 (95% CI, 0.94 to 1.20); prostate cancer RR, 1.06 (95% CI, 0.91 to 1.23); colorectal cancer RR, 1.44 (95% CI, 1.09 to 1.90).
†Subsequent ATBC publications after the initial publication[59] reclassified cancer cases: three additional prostate cancer cases were identified and seven were reclassified as nonmalignant; colorectal cancer cases excluded six participants with carcinoids and squamous cell carcinoma of the anal canal, an additional eight colorectal cancer cases were reclassified based on pathology.
‡Combined colon and rectal cancer cases.
§Total number of deaths during 6-year posttrial period only (excludes supplementation period).
∥Not cumulative; incidence during posttrial followup periods only (11 years: May 1993 to April 1996; 14 years: May 1996 to April 1999).

Abbreviations: ATBC = Alpha-Tocopherol Beta-Carotene Cancer Prevention; CARET = Carotene and Retinol Efficacy Trial; CI = confidence interval; NR = not reported; NSCPS = Nambour Skin Cancer Prevention Study; PHS-I = Physician's Health Study I; RR = relative risk; SCPS = Skin Cancer Prevention Study; WHS = Women's Health Study; y = years.

Table 16. All-Cause Mortality Among Beta-Carotene Studies

Study	Comparison	Mean followup (y)	Intervention, # of deaths (%)	Comparator, # of deaths (%)	RR	95% CI	P-value
SCPS[63,75]	Beta-carotene vs. placebo	5	79/913 (8.7)	72/892 (8.1)	1.08	0.98 to 1.19	NR
		8.2	146/913 (16)	139/892 (15.6)	1.03	0.82 to 1.30	0.80
NSCPS[64]	Beta-carotene vs. placebo	4.5	11/820 (1.3)	21/801 (2.6)	NR	NR	NR
PHS-I[61]	Beta-carotene vs. no beta-carotene	12	979/11,036 (8.9)	968/11,035 (8.8)	1.02	0.93 to 1.11	0.68
WHS[62]	Beta-carotene vs. no beta-carotene	4.1	59/19,937 (0.3)	55/19,939 (0.3)	1.07	0.74 to 1.56	0.70
ATBC†[59,73]	Beta-carotene vs. no beta-carotene	6.1	1,851/14,560 (12.7)	1,719/14,573 (11.8)	1.08	1.01 to 1.16	0.02
		8	1,851/14,560 (12.7)	1,719/14,573 (11.8)	1.08	1.01 to 1.15	NR
		11§	1,278/12,709 (10.1)	1,164/12,914 (9)	1.11	1.03 to 1.21	NR
		14§	1,455/11,431 (12.7)	1,401/11,690 (12)	1.07	0.99 to 1.15	NR
		16§	971/9,976 (9.7)	992/10,289 (9.6)	1.01	0.92 to 1.10	NR
CARET[60,74]	Beta-carotene + vitamin A vs. placebo	4	NR	NR	1.17*	1.03 to 1.33	0.02
		6‡	1,225/8,744 (14)	1,047/8,396 (12.5)	1.08*	0.99 to 1.17	0.07

*Unadjusted.
†Overall 6-year posttrial mortality rate was also statistically significant (RR, 1.07 [95% CI, 1.02 to 1.12]).[73]
‡Total number of deaths during 6-year posttrial period only (excludes supplementation period).
§Not cumulative; incidence during posttrial followup periods only (11 years: May 1993 to April 1996; 14 years: May 1996 to April 1999; 16 years: May 1999 to April 2001).

Abbreviations: ATBC = Alpha-Tocopherol Beta-Carotene Cancer Prevention; CARET = Carotene and Retinol Efficacy Trial; CI = confidence interval; NR = not reported; NSCPS = Nambour Skin Cancer Prevention Study; PHS-I = Physician's Health Study I; RR = relative risk; SCPS = Skin Cancer Prevention Study; WHS = Women's Health Study; y = years.

Table 17. Yellowing of the Skin Among Beta-Carotene Studies

Study	Comparison	Mean followup (y)	# of events among participants receiving beta-carotene (%)	# of events among participants not receiving beta-carotene (%)
ATBC[59]	Beta-carotene vs. no beta-carotene	6.1	4,950/14,560 (34)	1,020/14,573 (7)
PHS-I[61]	Beta-carotene vs. no beta-carotene	12	1,745/11,036 (15.8)	1,535/11,035 (13.9)
WHS[62]	Beta-carotene vs. no beta-carotene	4.1	2,131/19,937 (10.7)	1,944/19,939 (9.7)
SCPS[63]*	Beta-carotene vs. placebo	5	12/913 (1.3)	0/892 (0)
CARET†[60]	Beta-carotene + vitamin A vs. placebo	4	28/9,420 (0.3)	NR

*Reported among participants who stopped taking the study capsules due to capsule-related symptoms.
†Skin yellowing of grade 3 or higher (grade 1 representing normal or no symptoms; grades 4–5 representing severe symptoms).

Abbreviations: ATBC = Alpha-Tocopherol Beta-Carotene Cancer Prevention; CARET = Carotene and Retinol Efficacy Trial; NR = not reported; PHS-I = Physician's Health Study I; SCPS = Skin Cancer Prevention Study; WHS = Women's Health Study; y = years.

Table 18. Vitamin E Evidence Summary

Study Quality	Study design Followup (max)	Supplement and dose Supplement duration	N	Mean age (y)	% Female	CVD incidence	Cancer incidence	Mortality	Harms	Comments
ATBC[59,66,69-73,76, 78,87,88,155-157] Good	2x2 factorial RCT 16 years	Vitamin E 50 mg qd (alone or in combination with beta-carotene 20 mg qd) 6.1 years (mean) (range, 5 to 8 years)	29,133	57	0	NA	Any: ↔ Lung: ↔ CRC: ↔ Prostate: ↓‡ Breast: NA Other: ↔	↔	↔	
ASAP[79] Fair	2x2 factorial RCT 3 years	Vitamin E 91 mg bid (alone or in combination with vitamin C 250 mg bid) 3 years	520	60	51	NA	NA	↔	↔	
PHS-II[80,83,154] Good	2x2x2x2 factorial RCT 8 years	Vitamin E 400 IU qd (alone or in combination with beta-carotene, vitamin C, and/or MVI) 8 years (median)	14,641	64	0	Any: ↔ Stroke: ↔ MI: ↔	Any: ↔ Lung: ↔ CRC: ↔ Prostate: ↔ Breast: NA Other: ↔	↔	↔	Hemorrhagic stroke (↑)
WHS[81,165] Good	2x2x2 factorial RCT 10.1 years	Vitamin E 600 IU qod (alone or in combination with beta-carotene 50 mg qod or aspirin) 10.1 years (mean) (range, 8.2 to 10.9 years)	39,876	55	100	Any: ↔ Stroke: ↔ MI: ↔	Any: ↔ Lung: ↔ CRC: ↔ Prostate: NA Breast: ↔ Other: ↔	↔	↔	CVD death (↓); mixed bleeding adverse effects: hematuria (↔), gastrointestinal bleeding (↔), bruising (↔), and epistaxis (↑)
Graat 2002[52] Good	2x2 factorial RCT 1.3 years	Vitamin E 200 mg qd (alone or in combination with MVI) 1.3 years	652	73	50	NA	NA	NA	↔	Respiratory infections (↔)
SELECT[82,86,143, 166-171] Good	RCT 12 years	Vitamin E 400 IU qd (alone or in combination with selenium 200 mcg qd) 5.46 years (median) (range, 7 to 12 years)	35,533	63	0	Any: ↔ Stroke: NR MI: NR	Any: ↔ Lung: ↔ CRC: ↔ Prostate: ↑† Breast: NA Other: ↔	↔	↔	

†Increasing risk with longer followup (i.e., >5 years) in vitamin E alone intervention group.
‡Including prostate cancer deaths.

Abbreviations: ASAP = Antioxidant Supplementations in Atherosclerosis Prevention; ATBC = Alpha-Tocopherol Beta-Carotene Cancer Prevention; bid = twice daily; CRC = colorectal cancer; CVD = cardiovascular disease; MI = myocardial infarction; MVI = multivitamin; NA = not applicable; NR = not reported; PHS-II =

Table 18. Vitamin E Evidence Summary

Physician's Health Study II; qd = once daily; qod = every other day; RCT = randomized, controlled trial; SELECT = Selenium and Vitamin E Cancer Prevention Trial; WHS = Women's Health Study; y = year.

Legend: ↑ (statistically significant increase in risk of outcome from supplementation), ↔ (no statistically significant difference between intervention groups), ↓ (statistically significant decrease in risk of outcome from supplementation).

Table 19. Cardiovascular Disease Incidence and Mortality Among Vitamin E Studies

Outcome	Study	Comparison	Mean followup (y)	Intervention, # of subjects with events (%)	Comparator, # of subjects with events (%)	RR or HR	95% CI	P-value
Any CVD incidence	SELECT[82]‡	Vitamin E vs. placebo	5	1,034/8,737 (11.8)	1,050/8,696 (12.1)	0.98*	0.88 to 1.09†	NR
		Vitamin E + selenium vs. placebo	5	1,041/8,703 (12)	1,050/8,696 (12.1)	0.99*	0.89 to 1.10†	NR
	PHS-II[80]¶	Vitamin E vs. no vitamin E	8	620/7,315 (8.5)	625/7,326 (8.5)	1.01*	0.90 to 1.13	0.86
	WHS[81]	Vitamin E vs. no vitamin E	10.1	482/19,937 (2.4)	517/19,939 (2.6)	0.93	0.82 to 1.05	0.26
CHF incidence	PHS-II[80]	Vitamin E vs. no vitamin E	8	289/7,315 (4)	294/7,326 (4)	1.02*	0.87 to 1.20	0.80
	WHS[165]	Vitamin E vs. no vitamin E	10.1	106/19,913 (0.5)	114/19,902 (0.6)	0.93*	0.71 to 1.21	0.59
MI incidence	PHS-II[80]‖	Vitamin E vs. no vitamin E	8	240/7,315 (3.3)	271/7,326 (3.7)	0.90*	0.75 to 1.07	0.22
	WHS[81]	Vitamin E vs. no vitamin E	10.1	196/19,937 (1)	195/19,939 (1)	1.01	0.82 to 1.23	0.96
Stroke incidence	PHS-II[80]‖‡	Vitamin E vs. no vitamin E	8	327/7,315 (4.5)	227/7,326 (3.1)	1.07*	0.89 to 1.29	0.45
	WHS[81]‡	Vitamin E vs. no vitamin E	10.1	241/19,937 (1.2)	246/19,939 (1.2)	0.98	0.82 to 1.17	0.82
	SELECT[82]§	Vitamin E vs. placebo	5	70/8,737 (0.8)	92/8,696 (1)	NR	NR	NR
		Vitamin E + selenium vs. placebo	5	99/8,703 (1.1)	92/8,696 (1)	NR	NR	NR
Angina incidence	PHS-II[80]	Vitamin E vs. no vitamin E	8	689/7,315 (9.4)	736/7,326 (10)	0.94*	0.85 to 1.05	NR
Any CVD death	SELECT[82]‡	Vitamin E vs. placebo	5	119/8,737 (1.4)	142/8,696 (1.6)	0.84*	0.61 to 1.15†	NR
		Vitamin E + selenium vs. placebo	5	117/8,703 (1.3)	142/8,696 (1.6)	0.82*	0.60 to 1.13†	NR
	PHS-II[80]	Vitamin E vs. no vitamin E	8	258/7,315 (3.5)	251/7,326 (3.4)	1.07*	0.90 to 1.28	0.43
	WHS[81]	Vitamin E vs. no vitamin E	10.1	106/19,937 (0.5)	140/19,939 (0.7)	0.76	0.59 to 0.98	0.03
Fatal MI	PHS-II[80]	Vitamin E vs. no vitamin E	8	22/7,315 (0.3)	30/7,326 (0.4)	0.75*	0.43 to 1.31	NR
	WHS[81]	Vitamin E vs. no vitamin E	10.1	12/19,937 (0.1)	14/19,939 (1)	0.86	0.40 to 1.85	0.70
Fatal stroke	PHS-II[80]	Vitamin E vs. no vitamin E	8	45/7,315 (0.6)	56/7,326 (0.8)	0.86*	0.58 to 1.27	NR
	WHS[81]	Vitamin E vs. no vitamin E	10.1	21/19,937 (0.1)	24/19,939 (0.1)	0.88	0.49 to 1.57	0.66

*HR; SELECT was adjusted for age, sex, and smoking status at baseline.
†99% CI.
‡ Includes CVD-related deaths; nonfatal strokes and other nonfatal CVD events also reported.
§ Number of events and the HR for hemorrhagic, ischemic, and unspecified stroke type also reported.
‖ Nonfatal and fatal events.
¶ Includes nonfatal MI, nonfatal stroke, and CVD deaths.

Abbreviations: CHF = coronary heart failure; CI = confidence interval; CVD = cardiovascular disease; HR = hazard ratio; MI = myocardial infarction; NR = not reported; PHS-II = Physician's Health Study II; RR = relative risk; SELECT = Selenium and Vitamin E Cancer Prevention Trial; WHS = Women's Health Study; y = years.

Table 20. Cancer Incidence and Mortality Among Vitamin E Studies

Outcome	Study	Comparison	Mean followup (y)	Intervention, # of subjects with events (%)	Comparator, # of subjects with events (%)	RR or HR	95% CI	P-value
All cancer sites incidence	SELECT[82]	Vitamin E vs. placebo	5	856/8,737 (9.8)	824/8,696 (9.5)	1.03*	0.91 to 1.17‡	NR
			12	1,190/8,737 (13.6)	1,108/8,696 (12.7)	1.07*	0.96 to 1.19‡	0.13
		Vitamin E + selenium vs. placebo	5	846/8,703 (9.7)	824/8,696 (9.5)	1.02*	0.90 to 1.16†	NR
			12	1,149/8,703 (13.2)	1,108/8,696 (12.7)	1.02*	0.92 to 1.14†	0.60
	PHS-II[83]	Vitamin E vs. no vitamin E	8	984/7,315 (13)	959/7,326 (13)	1.04*	0.95 to 1.13	0.41
	WHS[81]	Vitamin E vs. no vitamin E	10.1	1,437/19,937 (7.2)	1,428/19,939 (7.2)	1.01	0.94 to 1.08	0.87
Lung cancer incidence	SELECT[82]	Vitamin E vs. placebo	5	67/8,737 (0.8)	67/8,696 (0.8)	1.00*	0.64 to 1.55‡	NR
			12	104/8,737 (1.2)	92/8,696 (1.1)	1.11*	0.76 to 1.61‡	0.49
		Vitamin E + selenium vs. placebo	5	78/8,703 (0.9)	67/8,696 (0.8)	1.16*	0.76 to 1.78†	NR
			12	104/8,703 (1.2)	92/8,696 (1.1)	1.11*	0.76 to 1.62†	0.48
	ATBC[59,73,¶]	Vitamin E vs. no vitamin E	6.1	433/14,564 (3)	443/14,569 (3)	1.02	NR	0.8
			8	444/14,564 (3)	451/14,569 (3.1)	0.99	0.87 to 1.12	NR
			11†	238/12,627 (1.9)	260/12,656 (2.1)	0.92	0.77 to 1.09	NR
			14†	287/11,431 (2.5)	252/11,405 (2.2)	1.14	0.96 to 1.35	NR
	PHS-II[83]	Vitamin E vs. no vitamin E	8	48/7,315 (0.7)	55/7,326 (0.8)	0.89*	0.60 to 1.31	0.55
	WHS[81]	Vitamin E vs. no vitamin E	10.1	107/19,937 (0.5)	98/19,939 (0.5)	1.09	0.83 to 1.44	0.52
Prostate cancer incidence	SELECT[82]	Vitamin E vs. placebo	5	473/8,737 (5.4)	416/8,696 (4.8)	1.13*	0.99 to 1.29	0.06
			12	620/8,737 (7.1)	529/8,696 (6.1)	1.17*	1.04 to 1.36‡	0.008
		Vitamin E + selenium vs. placebo	5	437/8,703 (5)	416/8,696 (4.8)	1.05*	0.91 to 1.20†	0.52
			12	555/8,703 (6.4)	529/8,696 (6.1)	1.05*	0.89 to 1.22†	0.46
	ATBC[59,73,76,¶]	Vitamin E vs. no vitamin E	6.1	99/14,564 (0.7)	147/14,569 (1)	0.68	0.44 to 0.94	0.002
			8	99/14,564 (0.7)	149/14,569 (1)	0.66	0.52 to 0.86	NR
			11†	130/12,696 (1)	147/12,694 (1.2)	0.89	0.70 to 1.12	NR
			14†	185/11,410 (1.6)	210/11,360 (1.8)	0.88	0.72 to 1.07	NR
	PHS-II[83]	Vitamin E vs. no vitamin E	8	493/7,315 (6.7)	515/7,326 (7)	0.97*	0.85 to 1.09	0.58
Breast cancer incidence	WHS[81]	Vitamin E vs. no vitamin E	10.1	616/19,937 (3.1)	614/19,939 (3.1)	1.00	0.90 to 1.12	0.95
Colorectal cancer incidence	SELECT[82]	Vitamin E vs. placebo	5	66/8,737 (0.8)	60/8,696 (0.7)	1.09*	0.69 to 1.73‡	NR
			12	85/8,737 (1.0)	75/8,696 (0.9)	1.09*	0.72 to 1.64‡	0.60
		Vitamin E + selenium vs. placebo	5	77/8,703 (0.9)	60/8,696 (0.7)	1.28*	0.82 to 2.00†	NR
			12	93/8,703 (1.1)	75/8,696 (0.9)	1.21*	0.81 to 1.81†	0.22
	ATBC[59,73,77]	Vitamin E vs. no vitamin E	6.1	59/14,564 (0.4)	76/14,569 (0.5)	0.78	0.55 to 1.09	NSD
			8	59/14,564 (0.4)	76/14,569 (0.5)	0.78	0.55 to 1.09	NR
			11†	50/12,733 (0.4)	42/12,756 (0.3)	1.19	0.79 to 1.80	NR
			14†	57/11,521 (0.5)	56/11,483 (0.5)	1.02	0.70 to 1.47	NR
	PHS-II[83]	Vitamin E vs. no vitamin E	8	75/7,315 (1)	87/7,326 (1.2)	0.88*	0.64 to 1.19	0.40
	WHS[81]	Vitamin E vs. no vitamin E	10.1	129/19,937 (0.6)	140/19,939 (0.7)	NR	NR	NR

Table 20. Cancer Incidence and Mortality Among Vitamin E Studies

Outcome	Study	Comparison	Mean followup (y)	Intervention, # of subjects with events (%)	Comparator, # of subjects with events (%)	RR or HR	95% CI	P-value
Any cancer death	SELECT[82]	Vitamin E vs. placebo	5	106/8,737 (1.2)	125/8,696 (1.4)	0.84*	0.60 to 1.18‡	NR
		Vitamin E + selenium vs. placebo	5	117/8,703 (1.3)	125/8,696 (1.4)	0.93*	0.67 to 1.30†	NR
	PHS-II[80]	Vitamin E vs. no vitamin E	8	273/7,315 (3.7)	250/7,326 (3.4)	1.13*	0.95 to 1.34	0.16
	WHS[81]	Vitamin E vs. no vitamin E	10.1	308/19,937 (1.5)	275/19,939 (1.4)	1.12	0.95 to 1.32	0.17
Lung cancer death	SELECT[82]	Vitamin E vs. placebo	5	38/8,737 (0.4)	41/8,696 (0.5)	0.92*	0.52 to 1.65‡	NR
		Vitamin E + selenium vs. placebo	5	39/8,703 (0.4)	41/8,696 (0.5)	0.95*	0.53 to 1.69†	NR
	ATBC[59,73]	Vitamin E vs. no vitamin E	6.1	285/14,564 (2)	279/14,569 (1.9)	NR	NR	NR
			12.1	942/5,298§ (17.8)		NR	NR	NR
	PHS-II[80]	Vitamin E vs. no vitamin E	8	44/7,315 (0.6)	43/7,326 (0.6)	1.05*	0.69 to 1.60	NR
Prostate cancer death	SELECT[82]	Vitamin E vs. placebo	5	0/8,737 (0)	0/8,696 (0)	NA	NA	NA
		Vitamin E + selenium vs. placebo	5	0/8,703 (0)	0/8,696 (0)	NA	NA	NA
	ATBC[76]	Vitamin E vs. no vitamin E	6.1	23/14,564 (0.2)	39/14,569 (0.3)	0.59	0.35 to 0.99	NR
	PHS-II[80]	Vitamin E vs. no vitamin E	8	37/7,315 (0.5)	39/7,326 (0.5)	1.01*	0.64 to 1.58	NR
Colorectal cancer death	SELECT[82]	Vitamin E vs. placebo	5	13/8,737 (0.1)	10/8,696 (0.1)	1.30*	0.44 to 3.83‡	NR
		Vitamin E + selenium vs. placebo	5	15/8,703 (0.2)	10/8,696 (0.1)	1.49*	0.52 to 4.28†	NR
	ATBC[77]	Vitamin E vs. no vitamin E	6.1	22/14,564 (0.2)	14/14,569 (0.1)	0.92	0.51 to 1.64	NR
	PHS-II[80]	Vitamin E vs. no vitamin E	8	21/7,315 (0.3)	32/7,326 (0.4)	0.68*	0.39 to 1.18	NR

*HR reported.
†Not cumulative; incidence during posttrial followup periods only (11 years: May 1993 to April 1996; 14 years: May 1996 to April 1999).
‡99% CI.
‖Subsequent ATBC publications after the initial publication[59] reclassified cancer cases: three additional prostate cancer cases were identified and seven were reclassified as nonmalignant; colorectal cancer cases excluded six participants with carcinoids and squamous cell carcinoma of the anal canal, an additional eight colorectal cancer cases were reclassified based on pathology.
¶Overall 6-year posttrial followup: lung cancer RR, 1.03 (95% CI, 0.91 to 1.16); prostate cancer RR, 0.88 (95% CI, 0.76 to 1.03).
§Total number of deaths during 6-year posttrial period.

Abbreviations: ATBC = Alpha-Tocopherol Beta-Carotene Cancer Prevention; CI = confidence interval; HR = hazard ratio; NR = not reported; PHS-II = Physician's Health Study II; RR = relative risk; SELECT = Selenium and Vitamin E Cancer Prevention Trial; WHS = Women's Health Study; y = years.

Table 21. All-Cause Mortality Among Vitamin E Studies

Study	Comparison	Mean followup (y)	Intervention, # of deaths (%)	Comparator, # of deaths (%)	RR or HR	95% CI	P-value
SELECT[82]	Vitamin E vs. placebo	5	358/8,737 (4.1)	382/8,696 (4.4)	0.93*	0.77 to 1.13‡	NR
		12	571/8,737 (6.5)	564/8,696 (6.5)	1.01*	0.86 to 1.17‡	0.91
	Vitamin E + selenium vs. placebo	5	359/8,703 (4.2)	382/8,696 (4.4)	0.94*	0.77 to 1.13‡	NR
		12	542/8,703 (6.2)	564/8,696 (6.5)	0.96*	0.82 to 1.12‡	0.47
ASAP[79]	Vitamin E vs. placebo	3	3/130 (2.3)	1/130 (0.8)	NR	NR	NR
	Vitamin E + vitamin C vs. placebo	3	1/130 (0.8)	1/130 (0.8)	NR	NR	NR
ATBC[59,73]	Vitamin E vs. no vitamin E	6.1	1,800/14,564 (12.4)	1,760/14,569 (12.1)	1.02	0.95 to 1.09	0.6
		8	1,800/14,564 (12.4)	1,770/14,569 (12.1)	1.02	0.95 to 1.09	NR
		11†	1,193/12,764 (9.3)	1,249/12,799 (9.8)	0.96	0.89 to 1.04	NR
		14†	1,460/11,571 (12.6)	1,396/11,550 (12.1)	1.05	0.97 to 1.13	NR
		16†	980/10,111 (9.7)	983/10,154 (9.7)	1.00	0.92 to 1.10	NR
PHS-II[80]	Vitamin E vs. no vitamin E	8	841/7,315 (11.5)	820/7,326 (11.2)	1.08*	0.98 to 1.19	0.13
WHS[81]	Vitamin E vs. no vitamin E	10.1	636/19,937 (3.2)	615/19,939 (3.1)	1.04	0.93 to 1.16	0.53

*HR.
†Not cumulative; incidence during posttrial followup periods only (11 years: May 1993 to April 1996; 14 years: May 1996 to April 1999; 16 years: May 1999 to April 2001).
‡99% CI.

Abbreviations: ASAP = Antioxidant Supplementations in Atherosclerosis Prevention; ATBC = Alpha-Tocopherol Beta-Carotene Cancer Prevention; CI = confidence interval; HR = hazard ratio; NR = not reported; PHS-II = Physician's Health Study II; RR = relative risk; SELECT = Selenium and Vitamin E Cancer Prevention Trial; WHS = Women's Health Study; y = years.

Table 22. Selenium Evidence Summary

Study Quality	Study design Followup (max)	Supplement and dose Supplement duration	N	Mean age (y)	% Female	CVD incidence	Cancer incidence	Mortality	Harms	Comments
NPC[89,90,92-95,172,173] Fair	RCT 7.6 years	Selenium 200 mcg qd 4.5 years (mean)	1,312	63	25	Any: ↔ MI: ↔ Stroke: ↔	Any: ↓ Lung: ↔ CRC: ↓ Prostate: ↓ Breast: ↔ Other: ↔	↔	↔	Cancer-related mortality (↓)
SELECT[82,86,143,166-171] Good	RCT 5 years with extended followup	Selenium 200 mcg qd (alone or in combination with vitamin E 400 IU qd) 5.46 years (median) (range, 7 to 12 years)	35,533	63	0	Any: ↔ MI: NR Stroke: NR	Any: ↔ Lung: ↔ CRC: ↔ Prostate: ↔ Breast: NA Other: ↔	↔	↑	Mixed dermatological harms among arms: selenium alone (↑) and selenium + vitamin E (↔)
U.K. PRECISE[91] Fair	RCT 0.5 years	Selenium 100, 200, or 300 mcg qd 0.5 years	501	67	47	NA	NA	NA	↔	No serious harms reported; stomach and abdominal discomfort (↔)

Abbreviations: CRC = colorectal cancer; CVD = cardiovascular disease; max = maximum; MI = myocardial infarction; NA = not applicable; NPC = Nutritional Prevention of Cancer; NR = not reported; qd = once daily; RCT = randomized, controlled trial; SELECT = Selenium and Vitamin E Cancer Prevention Trial; U.K. PRECISE = U.K. Prevention of Cancer by Intervention with Selenium; y = year.

Legend: ↑ (statistically significant increase in risk of outcome from supplementation), ↔ (no statistically significant difference between intervention groups), ↓ (statistically significant decrease in risk of outcome from supplementation).

Table 23. Cardiovascular Disease Incidence and Mortality Among Selenium Studies

Outcome	Study	Comparison	Mean followup (y)	Intervention, # of subjects with events (%)	Comparator, # of subjects with events (%)	RR or HR	95% CI	P-value
Any CVD incidence	NPC[173]	Selenium vs. placebo	7.6	103/504 (20.4)	96/500 (19.2)	1.03*	0.78 to 1.37	0.81
	SELECT[82]†	Selenium vs. placebo	5	1,080/8,752 (12.3)	1,050/8,696 (12.1)	1.02‖	0.92 to 1.13‡	NR
		Selenium + vitamin E vs. placebo		1,041/8,703 (12)	1,050/8,696 (12.1)	0.99	0.89 to 1.10‡	NR
Coronary heart disease incidence	NPC[173]	Selenium vs. placebo	7.6	63/500 (12.5)	59/500 (11.8)	1.04*	0.73 to 1.49	0.81
Cerebrovascular events incidence	NPC[173]	Selenium vs. placebo	7.6	40/504 (7.9)	37/500 (7.4)	1.02*	0.65 to 1.59	0.94
MI incidence	NPC[173]	Selenium vs. placebo	7.6	41/504 (8.1)	43/500 (8.6)	0.94*	0.61 to 1.44	0.77
Stroke incidence	NPC[173]	Selenium vs. placebo	7.6	35/504 (6.9)	32/500 (6.4)	1.02*	0.63 to 1.65	0.92
	SELECT[82]¶	Selenium vs. placebo	5	73/8,752 (0.8)	92/8,696 (1)	NR	NR	NR
		Vitamin E + selenium vs. placebo	5	99/8,703 (1.1)	92/8,696 (1)	NR	NR	NR
Any CVD death	NPC[89,92,173]	Selenium vs. placebo	6	47/653 (7.2)	46/659 (7)	1.00	0.66 to 1.55	0.96
	SELECT[82]§	Selenium vs. placebo	7.6	40/504 (7.9)	31/500 (6.2)	1.22*	0.76 to 1.95	0.41
		Selenium vs. placebo	5	129/8,752 (1.5)	142/8,696 (1.6)	0.91‖	0.66 to 1.24	NR
		Selenium + vitamin E vs. placebo		117/8,703 (1.3)	142/8,696 (1.6)	0.82*	0.60 to 1.13†	NR
Fatal MI	NPC[173]	Selenium vs. placebo	7.6	9/504 (1.8)	8/500 (1.6)	1.05*	0.42 to 2.80	0.88

*HR; adjusted for age, sex, and smoking status at baseline.
†Includes CVD-related deaths; nonfatal strokes and other nonfatal CVD events also reported.
‡99% CI reported.
§Fatal hemorrhagic stroke and other fatal CVD events (not specified) also reported.
‖HR; analyses did not incorporate adjustments for baseline covariates.
¶Number of events and the HR for hemorrhagic, ischemic, and unspecified stroke type also reported.

Abbreviations: CI = confidence interval; CVD = cardiovascular disease; HR = hazard ratio; MI = myocardial infarction; NR = not reported; NPC = Nutritional Prevention of Cancer; RR = relative risk; SELECT = Selenium and Vitamin E Cancer Prevention Trial; y = years.

Table 24. Cancer Incidence and Mortality Among Selenium Studies

Outcome	Study	Comparison	Mean followup (y)	Intervention, # of subjects with events (%)	Comparator, # of subjects with events (%)	RR‡ or HR	95% CI	P-value
Any cancer incidence	NPC[89,92]	Selenium vs. placebo	6	77/653 (11.8)	119/659 (18.1)	0.63	0.47 to 0.85	0.001
			7.4	105/621 (16.9)	137/629 (21.8)	0.75	0.58 to 0.98	0.03
	SELECT[82]	Selenium vs. placebo	5	837/8,752 (9.6)	824/8,696 (9.5)	1.01*	0.89 to 1.15†	NR
			12	1,132/8,752 (12.9)	1,108/8,696 (12.7)	1.02*	0.92 to 1.14†	0.59
		Selenium + vitamin E vs. placebo	5	846/8,703 (9.7)	824/8,696 (9.5)	1.02*	0.90 to 1.16†	NR
			12	1,149/8,703 (13.2)	1,108/8,696 (12.7)	1.02*	0.92 to 1.14†	0.60
Prostate cancer incidence	NPC[89,90,92,93,95]	Selenium vs. placebo	6	13/470 (2.7)	35/495 (7.1)	0.37	0.18 to 0.71	0.002
			7.4	22/457 (4.8)	42/470 (8.9)	0.51	0.29 to 0.88	0.009
	SELECT[82]	Selenium vs. placebo	5	432/8,752 (4.9)	416/8,696 (4.8)	1.04*	0.90 to 1.18†	0.62
			12	575/8,752 (6.6)	529/8,696 (6.1)	1.09*	0.93 to 1.27†	0.18
		Selenium + vitamin E vs. placebo	5	437/8,703 (5)	416/8,696 (4.8)	1.05*	0.91 to 1.20†	0.52
			12	555/8,703 (6.4)	529/8,696 (6.1)	1.05*	0.89 to 1.22†	0.46
Lung cancer incidence	NPC[89,90,92,94]	Selenium vs. placebo	6	17/653 (2.6)	31/659 (4.7)	0.54	0.30 to 0.98	0.04
			7.4	25/621 (4)	35/629 (5.6)	0.70	0.40 to 1.21	0.18
	SELECT[82]	Selenium vs. placebo	5	75/8,752 (0.9)	67/8,696 (0.8)	1.12*	0.73 to 1.72†	NR
			12	94/8,752 (1.1)	92/8,696 (1.1)	1.02*	0.70 to 1.50†	0.89
		Selenium + vitamin E vs. placebo	5	78/8,703 (0.9)	67/8,696 (0.8)	1.16*	0.76 to 1.78†	NR
			12	104/8,703 (1.2)	92/8,696 (1.1)	1.11*	0.76 to 1.62†	0.48
Colorectal cancer incidence	NPC[89,90,92]	Selenium vs. placebo	6.3	8/653 (1.2)	19/659 (2.9)	0.42	0.18 to 0.95	0.03
			7.4	9/621 (1.4)	19/629 (3)	0.46	0.19 to 1.08	0.055
	SELECT[82]	Selenium vs. placebo	5	63/8,752 (0.7)	60/8,696 (0.7)	1.05*	0.66 to 1.67†	NR
			12	74/8,752 (0.8)	75/8,696 (0.9)	0.96*	0.63 to 1.46†	0.79
		Selenium + vitamin E vs. placebo	5	77/8,703 (0.9)	60/8,696 (0.7)	1.28*	0.82 to 2.00†	NR
			12	93/8,703 (1.1)	75/8,696 (0.9)	1.21*	0.81 to 1.81†	0.22
Breast cancer incidence	NPC[89,90]	Selenium vs. placebo	6.3	9/653 (1.4)	3/659 (0.5)	2.88	0.72 to 16.5	0.09
			7.4	11/621 (1.8)	6/629 (1)	1.82	0.62 to 6.01	0.24
Any cancer death	NPC[89,90,92]	Selenium vs. placebo	6.3	29/653 (4.4)	57/659 (8.6)	0.50	0.31 to 0.80	0.002
			7.4	40/621 (6.4)	66/629 (10.5)	0.59	0.39 to 0.89	0.008
	SELECT[82]	Selenium vs. placebo	5	128/8,752 (1.5)	125/8,696 (1.4)	1.02*	0.74 to 1.41†	NR
		Selenium + vitamin E vs. placebo	5	117/8,703 (1.3)	125/8,696 (1.4)	0.93*	0.67 to 1.30†	NR
Lung cancer death	NPC[89,92]	Selenium vs. placebo	6	12/653 (1.8)	25/659 (3.8)	0.47	0.22 to 0.98	0.03
	SELECT[82]	Selenium vs. placebo	5	45/8,752 (6.9)	41/8,696 (6.2)	1.10*	0.63 to 1.91†	NR
		Selenium + vitamin E vs. placebo	5	39/8,703 (0.4)	41/8,696 (0.5)	0.95*	0.53 to 1.69†	NR
Prostate cancer death	SELECT[82]	Selenium vs. placebo	5	1/8,752 (0)	0/8,696 (0)	NA	NA	NA
		Selenium + vitamin E vs. placebo	5	0/8,703 (0)	0/8,696 (0)	NA	NA	NA

Table 24. Cancer Incidence and Mortality Among Selenium Studies

Outcome	Study	Comparison	Mean followup (y)	Intervention, # of subjects with events (%)	Comparator, # of subjects with events (%)	RR‡ or HR	95% CI	P-value
Colorectal cancer death	SELECT[32]	Selenium vs. placebo	5	10/8,752 (0.1)	10/8,696 (0.1)	1.00*	0.32 to 3.16†	NR
		Selenium + vitamin E vs. placebo	5	15/8,703 (0.2)	10/8,696 (0.1)	1.49*	0.52 to 4.28†	NR

*HR; analyses did not incorporate adjustments for baseline covariates.
†99% CI reported.
‡Unadjusted.

Abbreviations: CI = confidence interval; HR = hazard ratio; NA = not applicable; NPC = Nutritional Prevention of Cancer; NR = not reported; RR = relative risk; SELECT = Selenium and Vitamin E Cancer Prevention Trial; y = years.

Table 25. All-Cause Mortality Among Selenium Studies

Study	Comparison	Mean followup (y)	Intervention, # of deaths (%)	Comparator, # of deaths (%)	RR or HR	95% CI	P-value
NPC[89,92,173]	Selenium vs. placebo	6	108/653 (16.5)	129/659 (19.6)	0.83‡	0.63 to 1.08	0.14
		7.6	110/504 (21.8)	110/500 (22)	0.95§	0.73 to 1.24	0.71
SELECT[82]	Selenium vs. placebo	5	378/8,752 (4.3)	382/8,696 (4.4)	0.99*	0.82 to 1.19	NR
		12	551/8,752 (6.3)	564/8,696 (6.5)	0.98*	0.84 to 1.14	0.67
	Selenium + vitamin E vs. placebo	5	359/8,703 (4.2)	382/8,696 (4.4)	0.94*	0.77 to 1.13	NR
		12	542/8,703 (6.2)	564/8,696 (6.5)	0.96*	0.82 to 1.12	0.47

*HR; analyses did not incorporate adjustments for baseline covariates.
†Noncardiovascular mortality also reported.
‡Unadjusted.
§HR; adjusted for age, sex, and smoking status at baseline.
|| 99% CI reported.

Abbreviations: CI = confidence interval; HR = hazard ratio; NPC = Nutritional Prevention of Cancer; NR = not reported; RR = relative risk; SELECT = Selenium and Vitamin E Cancer Prevention Trial;y = years.

Table 26. Vitamin A Evidence Summary

Study Quality	Study design Followup (max)	Supplement and dose Supplement duration	N	Mean age (y)	% Female	CVD incidence	Cancer incidence	Mortality	Harms	Comments
SKICAP-AK[97,174] Fair	RCT 5 years	Vitamin A 25,000 IU qd 5 years	2,297	63	30	NA	NA	↔	↔	
SKICAP-S/B[98,174] Fair	RCT 3 years	Vitamin A 25,000 IU qd 3 years	347	NR	28	NA	NA	NA	↔	
CARET[60,67,74,161-164] Good	RCT 11 years	Vitamin A 25,000 IU qd + beta-carotene 30 mg qd NR	18,314	58	34	NA	Any: ↔ Lung: ↑* CRC: ↔ Prostate: ↔ Breast: ↔ Other: ↔	↑	↔	Baseline population at high risk for lung cancer (smokers or asbestos-exposed workers)
NHS[53] Good	Prospective cohort 18 years	Vitamin A users (dose NR) NR	72,337	58	100	NA	NA	NA	↑	Hip fracture among current (↔) and past (↑) vitamin A supplement users
IWHS[96] Good	Prospective cohort 9.5 years	Vitamin A users (dose NR) NR	34,703	61	100	NA	NA	NA	↔	All fractures (↔) and hip fractures (↔)

*Including lung cancer deaths.

Abbreviations: CARET = Carotene and Retinol Efficacy Trial; CRC = colorectal cancer; CVD = cardiovascular disease; IWHS = Iowa Women's Health Study; max = maximum; NA = not applicable; NHS = Nurses' Health Study; NR = not reported; qd = once daily; RCT = randomized, controlled trial; SKICAP-AK = Skin Cancer Prevention Trial-Actinic Keratoses; SKICAP-S/B = Skin Cancer Prevention Trial-Squamous/Basal Cell Carcinoma; y = years.

Legend: ↑ (statistically significant increase in risk of outcome from supplementation), ↔ (no statistically significant difference between intervention groups), ↓ (statistically significant decrease in risk of outcome from supplementation).

Table 27. Vitamin C Evidence Summary

Study Quality	Study design Followup	Supplement and dose Supplement duration	N	Mean age (y)	% Female	CVD incidence	Cancer incidence	Mortality	Harms	Comments
PHS-II[80,83,154] Good	2x2x2x2 factorial RCT 8 years	Vitamin C 500 mg qd (alone or in combination with vitamin E, beta-carotene, and/or MVI) 8 years (median)	14,641	64	0	Any: ↔ MI: ↔ Stroke: ↔	Any: ↔ Lung: ↔ CRC: ↔ Prostate: ↔ Breast: NA Other: ↔	↔	NR	
ASAP[79] Fair	2x2 factorial RCT 3 years	Vitamin C 250 mg bid (alone or combined with vitamin E 91 mg bid) 3 years	520	60	51	NA	NA	↔	↔	

Abbreviations: ASAP = Antioxidant Supplementations in Atherosclerosis Prevention; bid = twice daily; CRC = colorectal cancer; CVD = cardiovascular disease; MI = myocardial infarction; MVI = multivitamin; NA = not applicable; NR = not reported; PHS-II = Physician's Health Study II; qd = once daily; RCT = randomized, controlled trial; y = years.

Legend: ↑ (statistically significant increase in risk of outcome from supplementation), ↔ (no statistically significant difference between intervention groups), ↓ (statistically significant decrease in risk of outcome from supplementation).

Table 28. Cardiovascular Disease Incidence and Mortality Among Vitamin C Studies

Outcome	Study	Comparison	Mean followup (y)	Intervention, # of subjects with events (%)	Comparator, # of subjects with events (%)	HR†	95% CI	P-value
Any CVD incidence‡	PHS-II[30]	Vitamin C vs. no vitamin C	8	619/7,329 (8.4)	626/7,312 (8.6)	0.99	0.89 to 1.11	0.91
MI incidence§				260/7,329 (3.5)	251/7,312 (3.4)	1.04	0.87 to 1.24	0.65
Stroke incidence*				218/7,329 (3)	246/7,312 (3.4)	0.89	0.89 to 1.07	0.21
CHF incidence				293/7,329 (4)	290/7,312 (4)	1.02	0.87 to 1.20	NR
Angina incidence				686/7,329 (9.4)	739/7,312 (10.1)	0.92	0.97 to 1.18	NR
Any CVD death				256/7,329 (3.5)	253/7,312 (3.5)	1.02	0.85 to 1.21	0.86
Fatal MI				30/7,329 (0.4)	22/7,312 (0.3)	1.37	0.79 to 2.38	NR
Fatal stroke				44/7,329 (0.6)	57/7,312 (0.8)	0.77	0.52 to 1.14	NR

*Hemorrhagic and ischemic stroke also reported separately; includes fatal and nonfatal events.
†HRs adjusted for age, study cohort, and randomized assignment.
‡Includes nonfatal strokes, nonfatal MI, and CVD deaths.
§Includes fatal and nonfatal events.

Abbreviations: CHF = coronary heart failure; CI = confidence interval; CVD = cardiovascular disease; HR = hazard ratio; MI = myocardial infarction; NR = not reported; PHS-II = Physician's Health Study II; y = years.

Table 29. Cancer Incidence and Mortality Among Vitamin C Studies

Outcome	Study	Comparison	Mean followup (y)	Intervention, # of subjects with events (%)	Comparator, # of subjects with events (%)	HR*	95% CI	P-value
Any cancer incidence	PHS-II[83]	Vitamin C vs. no vitamin C	8	973/7,329 (13.3)	970/7,312 (13.3)	1.01	0.92 to 1.10	0.86
Lung cancer incidence				50/7,329 (0.7)	53/7,312 (0.7)	0.95	0.64 to 1.39	0.78
Prostate cancer incidence				508/7,329 (6.9)	500/7,312 (6.8)	1.02	0.90 to 1.15	0.80
Colorectal cancer incidence				75/7,329 (1)	87/7,312 (1.2)	0.86	0.63 to 1.17	0.35
Any cancer death				268/7,329 (3.7)	255/7,312 (3.5)	1.06	0.89 to 1.25	0.53
Lung cancer death				39/7,329 (0.5)	48/7,312 (0.7)	0.82	0.53 to 1.25	NR
Prostate cancer death				45/7,329 (0.6)	31/7,312 (0.4)	1.46	0.92 to 2.31	NR
Colorectal cancer death				27/7,329 (0.4)	26/7,312 (0.4)	1.04	0.61 to 1.78	NR

*HRs adjusted for age, study cohort, and randomized assignment.

Abbreviations: CI = confidence interval; HR = hazard ratio; NR = not reported; PHS-II = Physician's Health Study II; y = years.

Table 30. All-Cause Mortality Among Vitamin C Studies

Study	Comparison	Mean followup (y)	Intervention, # of deaths (%)	Comparator, # of deaths (%)	RR	95% CI	P-value
ASAP[79]	Vitamin C vs. placebo	3	1/130 (0.8)	1/130 (0.8)	NR	NR	NR
	Vitamin C + vitamin E vs. placebo	3	1/130 (0.8)	1/130 (0.8)	NR	NR	NR
PHS-II[80,83]	Vitamin C vs. no vitamin C	8	857/7,329 (11.7)	804/7,312 (11)	1.07*	0.97 to 1.18	0.17

*†Hazard ratio; adjusted for age, study cohort, and randomized assignment.

Abbreviations: ASAP = Antioxidant Supplementations in Atherosclerosis Prevention; CI = confidence interval; NR = not reported; PHS-II = Physician's Health Study II; RR = relative risk; y = years.

Table 31. Folic Acid Evidence Summary

Study Quality	Study design Followup (max)	Supplement and dose Supplement duration	N	Mean age (y)	% Female	CVD incidence	Cancer incidence	Mortality	Harms	Comments
AFPPS[101,102] Fair	3x2 factorial RCT 10 years	Folic acid 1 mg qd 3 years*	1,021	57	36	Any: ↔ MI: ↔ Stroke: ↔	Any: ↑ Lung: NR CRC: NA Prostate: ↑ Breast: NR Other: NR	↔	NR	Paradoxical effect for noncolorectal cancers (↑)

*Subjects invited to continue their random assignment (i.e., folic acid or placebo) for an additional 3 to 5 years after the initial 3-year followup examination; range of followup, 3 to 8 years.

Abbreviations: AFPPS = Aspirin/Folate Polyp Prevention Study; CRC = colorectal cancer; CVD = cardiovascular disease; max = maximum; MI = myocardial infarction; NA = not applicable; NR = not reported; qd = once daily; RCT = randomized, controlled trial; y = year.

Legend: ↑ (statistically significant increase in risk of outcome from supplementation), ↔ (no statistically significant difference between intervention groups), ↓ (statistically significant decrease in risk of outcome from supplementation).

Table 32. Vitamin D Evidence Summary

Study Quality	Study design Followup (max)	Supplement and dose Supplement duration	N	Mean age (y)	% Female	CVD incidence	Cancer incidence	Mortality	Harms	Comments
RECORD[103,106,107] Fair	2x2 factorial RCT 6.2 years	Vitamin D₃ 800 IU qd (alone or in combination with calcium 1,000 mg qd) 3.75 years (median) (range, 2 to 5.2 years)	5,292	77	85	Any: ↔ MI: ↔ Stroke: ↔	Any: ↔ Lung: ↔ CRC: ↔ Prostate: ↔ Breast: ↔ Other: ↔	↔	↔	
Trivedi 2003[104] Fair	RCT 5 years	Vitamin D₃ 100,000 IU every 4 months 5 years	2,686	75	24	Any: ↔ MI: NR Stroke: ↔	Any: ↔ Lung: ↔ CRC: ↔ Prostate: NR Breast: NR Other: NR	↔†	NR	
Dean, 2011[105] Good	RCT 0.1 years	Vitamin D 5,000 IU qd 0.1 years	128	22	57	NA	NA	NA	↔	

*CVD mortality only.
†Cancer and CVD-related mortality also reported; no significant difference between groups.

Abbreviations: bid = twice daily; CRC = colorectal cancer; CVD = cardiovascular disease; max = maximum; MI = myocardial infarction; NA = not applicable; NR = not reported; qd = once daily; RCT = randomized, controlled trial; RECORD = Randomized Evaluation of Calcium or Vitamin D; y = years.

Legend: ↑ (statistically significant increase in risk of outcome from supplementation), ↔ (no statistically significant difference between intervention groups), ↓ (statistically significant decrease in risk of outcome from supplementation).

Table 33. Cardiovascular Disease Incidence and Mortality Among Vitamin D Studies

Outcome	Study	Comparison	Mean followup (y)	Intervention, # of subjects with events (%)	Comparator, # of subjects with events (%)	RR or HR	95% CI	P-value
Any CVD incidence	Trivedi 2003§[104]	Vitamin D vs. placebo	5	477/1,345 (35.5)	503/1,341 (37.5)	0.90‡	0.77 to 1.06	0.22
	RECORD[105]	Vitamin D vs. no vitamin D	6.1	339/2,649 (12.8)	363/2,643 (13.7)	0.96†	0.82 to 1.13	0.61
Ischemic heart disease incidence	Trivedi 2003[104]	Vitamin D vs. placebo	5	224/1,345 (16.7)	233/1,341 (17.4)	0.94	0.77 to 1.15	0.57
Cerebrovascular disease incidence	Trivedi 2003[104]	Vitamin D vs. placebo	5	105/1,345 (7.8)	101/1,341 (7.5)	1.02	0.77 to 1.36	0.87
Cardiac failure incidence	RECORD[105]	Vitamin D vs. no vitamin D	6.1	102/2,649 (3.9)	136/2,643 (5.1)	0.73†	0.55 to 0.96	0.03
MI incidence	RECORD[105]	Vitamin D vs. no vitamin D	6.1	114/2,649 (4.3)	117/2,643 (4.4)	1.04†	0.79 to 1.37	0.76
Stroke incidence	RECORD[105]	Vitamin D vs. no vitamin D	6.1	160/2,649 (6.0)	149/2,643 (5.6)	1.13†	0.88 to 1.44	0.33
Any CVD death	Trivedi 2003[104]	Vitamin D vs. placebo	5	101/1,345 (7.5)	117/1,341 (8.7)	0.84	0.65 to 1.1	0.20
	RECORD[105]*	Vitamin D vs. no vitamin D	6.2	350/2,649 (13.2)	376/2,643 (14.2)	0.91†	0.79 to 1.05	0.175
Fatal ischemic heart disease	Trivedi 2003[104]	Vitamin D vs. placebo	5	42/1,345 (3.1)	49/1,341 (3.7)	0.84	0.56 to 1.27	0.41
Fatal CHD	RECORD[105]*	Vitamin D vs. no vitamin D	6.2	162/2,649 (6.1)	176/2,643 (6.7)	NR	NR	NR
Fatal stroke	Trivedi 2003[104]	Vitamin D vs. placebo	5	28/1,345 (2.1)	26/1,341 (1.9)	1.04	0.61 to 1.77	0.89
	RECORD[105]*	Vitamin D vs. no vitamin D	6.2	115/2,649 (4.3)	105/2,643 (4.0)	NR	NR	NR

*Deaths by other vascular diseases also reported.
†HR, unadjusted.
‡Adjusted for age.
§Self-reported incidence or when indicated as cause of death.

Abbreviations: CI = confidence interval; CHD = coronary heart disease; CVD = cardiovascular disease; HR = hazard ratio; MI = myocardial infarction; NR = not reported; RECORD = Randomized Evaluation of Calcium or Vitamin D; RR = relative risk; y = years.

Table 34. Cancer Incidence and Mortality Among Vitamin D Studies

Outcome	Study	Comparison	Mean followup (y)	Intervention, # of subjects with events (%)	Comparator, # of subjects with events (%)	RR or HR	95% CI	P-value
Any cancer incidence	Trivedi 2003[104]‡	Vitamin D vs. placebo	5	188/1,345 (14)	173/1,341 (12.9)	1.09†	0.86 to 1.36	0.47
	RECORD[103]	Vitamin D vs. no vitamin D	6.2	369/2,649 (13.9)	354/2,643 (13.4)	1.07*	0.92 to 1.25	0.376
Breast cancer incidence	RECORD[103]	Vitamin D vs. no vitamin D	6.2	43/2,649 (1.6)	37/2,643 (1.4)	NR	NR	NR
Colorectal cancer incidence	Trivedi 2003[104]§	Vitamin D vs. placebo	5	28/1,345 (2.1)	27/1,341 (2.0)	1.02	0.6 to 1.74	0.94
	RECORD[103]	Vitamin D vs. no vitamin D	6.2	41/2,649 (1.5)	30/2,643 (1.1)	NR	NR	NR
Lung cancer incidence	Trivedi 2003[104]‖	Vitamin D vs. placebo	5	17/1,345 (1.3)	15/1,341 (1.1)	1.12	0.56 to 2.25	0.75
	RECORD[103]	Vitamin D vs. no vitamin D	6.2	24/2,649 (0.9)	32/2,643 (1.2)	NR	NR	NR
Prostate cancer incidence	RECORD[103]	Vitamin D vs. no vitamin D	6.2	17/2,649 (0.6)	12/2,643 (0.5)	NR	NR	NR
Any cancer death	Trivedi 2003[104]	Vitamin D vs. placebo	5	63/1,345 (4.7)	72/1,341 (5.4)	0.86	0.61 to 1.2	0.37
	RECORD[103]	Vitamin D vs. no vitamin D	6.2	151/2,649 (5.7)	178/2,643 (6.7)	0.85*	0.68 to 1.06	0.157
Breast cancer death	RECORD[103]	Vitamin D vs. no vitamin D	6.2	14/2,649 (0.5)	13/2,643 (0.5)	NR	NR	NR
Colorectal cancer death	Trivedi 2003[104]§	Vitamin D vs. placebo	5	7/1,345 (0.5)	11/1,341 (0.8)	0.62	0.24 to 1.6	0.33
	RECORD[103]	Vitamin D vs. no vitamin D	6.2	20/2,649 (0.8)	13/2,643 (0.5)	NR	NR	NR
Lung cancer death	Trivedi 2003[104]‖	Vitamin D vs. placebo	5	10/1,345 (0.7)	11/1,341 (0.8)	0.89	0.38 to 2.09	0.78
	RECORD[103]	Vitamin D vs. no vitamin D	6.2	24/2,649 (0.9)	34/2,643 (1.3)	NR	NR	NR
Prostate cancer death	RECORD[103]	Vitamin D vs. no vitamin D	6.2	6/2,649 (0.2)	6/2,643 (0.2)	NR	NR	NR

*HR, unadjusted.
†RR adjusted by age.
‡Incidence number of cancers excluding skin cancer also reported; no significant difference between groups.
§Colon cancer only.
‖Respiratory cancers.

Abbreviations: CI = confidence interval; HR = hazard ratio; NR = not reported; RECORD = Randomized Evaluation of Calcium or Vitamin D; RR = relative risk; y = years.

Table 35. All-Cause Mortality Among Vitamin D Studies

Study	Comparison	Mean followup (y)	Intervention, # of deaths (%)	Comparator, # of deaths (%)	RR or HR	95% CI	P-value
Trivedi 2003[104]	Vitamin D vs. placebo	5	224/1,345 (16.7)	247/1,341 (18.4)	0.88†	0.74 to 1.06	0.18
RECORD[103]	Vitamin D vs. no vitamin D	6.2	836/2,649 (31.6)	881/2,643 (33.3)	0.93*	0.85 to 1.02	0.132

*HR; unadjusted.
†Adjusted for age.

Abbreviations: CI = confidence interval; HR = hazard ratio; NR = not reported; RECORD = Randomized Evaluation of Calcium or Vitamin D; RR = relative risk; y = years.

Table 36. Vitamin D and Calcium Evidence Summary

Study Quality	Study design Followup (max)	Supplement and dose Supplement duration	N	Mean age (y)	% Female	CVD incidence	Cancer incidence	Mortality	Harms	Comments
Lappe 2007[109,175] Fair	RCT 4 years	Vitamin D_3 25 mcg qd + calcium 1,400 mg qd 4 years	1,180	67	100	NR	Any: ↓ Lung: ↔ CRC: ↔ Prostate: NA Breast: ↔ Other: ↔	NR	↔	
WHI[108,110-112,137,176-185] Good	RCT 7 years	Vitamin D_3 200 IU bid + calcium 500 mg bid 7 years (mean)	36,282	62	100	Any: ↔ MI: ↔ Stroke: ↔	Any: ↔ Lung: NR CRC: ↔ Prostate: NA Breast: ↔ Other: ↔	↔	↑	Kidney stones (↑)

Abbreviations: bid = twice daily; CRC = colorectal cancer; CVD = cardiovascular disease; MI = myocardial infarction; NA = not applicable; NR = not reported; qd = once daily; RCT = randomized, controlled trial; WHI = Women's Health Initiative; y = years.

Legend: ↑ (statistically significant increase in risk of outcome from supplementation), ↔ (no statistically significant difference between intervention groups), ↓ (statistically significant decrease in risk of outcome from supplementation).

Table 37. Cardiovascular Disease Incidence and Mortality Among Combined Vitamin D and Calcium Supplement Studies

Outcome	Study	Comparison	Mean followup (y)	Intervention, # of subjects with events (%)	Comparator, # of subjects with events (%)	HR†	95% CI	P-value
Any CVD incidence‡	WHI[112,181,183]	Vitamin D + calcium vs. placebo	7	1,832/18,176 (10.1)	1,810/18,106 (10.0)	1.00	0.94 to 1.07	
Any heart disease incidence*				1,405/18,176 (7.7)	1,363/18,106 (7.5)	1.02	0.95 to 1.11	NR
CHD incidence||				499/18,176 (2.7)	475/18,106 (2.6)	1.03†	0.90 to 1.17	
MI incidence				411/18,176 (2.3)	390/18,106 (2.2)	1.05	0.91 to 1.20	0.52
Angina incidence				404/18,176 (2.2)	377/18,106 (2.1)	1.08	0.94 to 1.24	0.30
Stroke incidence§				362/18,176 (2)	377/18,106 (2.1)	0.95	0.82 to 1.10	0.51
Heart failure (hospital) incidence				394/18,176 (2.2)	407/18,106 (2.2)	0.95	0.83 to 1.10	0.50
TIA incidence				213/18,176 (1.2)	182/18,106 (1)	1.16	0.95 to 1.42	0.13
Any CVD death				226/18,176 (1.2)	244/18,106 (1.3)	0.92	0.77 to 1.10	NR
Fatal CHD				130/18,176 (0.7)	128/18,106 (0.7)	1.01	0.79 to 1.29	0.52
Fatal MI or CHD				499/18,176 (2.7)	475/18,106 (2.6)	1.04	0.92 to 1.18	NR

*Total heart disease includes CHD, revascularization, angina, and congestive heart failure.
†HR, unadjusted.
‡Total CVD includes total heart disease, stroke, carotid artery disease, and peripheral vascular disease.
§Ischemic, hemorrhagic, and other stroke also reported.
\|\| Included nonfatal MI and CHD death.

Abbreviations: CI = confidence interval; CHD = coronary heart disease; CVD = cardiovascular disease; HR = hazard ratio; MI = myocardial infarction; TIA = transient ischemic attack; WHI = Women's Health Initiative; y = years.

Table 38. Cancer Incidence and Mortality Among Combined Vitamin D and Calcium Supplement Studies

Outcome	Study	Comparison	Mean followup (y)	Intervention, # of subjects with events (%)	Comparator, # of subjects with events (%)	RR or HR	95% CI	P-value
Any cancer incidence	Lappe 2007[109]	Vitamin D + calcium vs. placebo	4	13/446 (2.9)	20/288 (6.9)	0.402	0.20 to 0.82	0.013
	WHI[108]	Vitamin D + calcium vs. placebo	7	1,634/18,176 (9.0)	1,655/18,106 (9.1)	0.98*	0.91 to 1.05	0.53
Breast cancer incidence	Lappe 2007[109]	Vitamin D + calcium vs. placebo	4	5/446 (1.1)	8/228 (2.8)	NR	NR	NR
	WHI[178]	Vitamin D + calcium vs. placebo	7	668/18,176 (3.7)	693/18,106 (3.8)	0.96*	0.86 to 1.07	NR
Colorectal cancer incidence	Lappe 2007[109]	Vitamin D + calcium vs. placebo	4	1/446 (0.2)	2/228 (0.9)	NR	NR	NR
	WHI[108]	Vitamin D + calcium vs. placebo	7	168/18,176 (0.9)	154/18,106 (0.9)	1.08*	0.86 to 1.34	0.51
Lung cancer incidence	Lappe 2007[109]	Vitamin D + calcium vs. placebo	4	1/446 (0.2)	3/228 (1.3)	NR	NR	NR
Any cancer death	WHI[108]	Vitamin D + calcium vs. placebo	7	344/18,176 (1.9)	385/18,106 (2.1)	0.89*	0.77 to 1.03	0.12
Breast cancer death	WHI[178]	Vitamin D + calcium vs. placebo	7	23/18,176 (0.1)	23/18,106 (0.1)	0.99*	0.55 to 1.76	NR
Colorectal cancer death	WHI[108]	Vitamin D + calcium vs. placebo	7	34/18,176 (0.2)	41/18,106 (0.2)	0.82*	0.52 to 1.29	0.39

*HR.

Abbreviations: CI = confidence interval; HR = hazard ratio; NR = not reported; RR = relative risk; WHI = Women's Health Initiative; y = years.

Table 39. All-Cause Mortality Among Combined Vitamin D and Calcium Supplement Studies

Study	Comparison	Mean followup (y)	Intervention, # of deaths (%)	Comparator, # of deaths (%)	HR*	95% CI	P-value
WHI[108]	Vitamin D + calcium vs. placebo	7	744/18,176 (4.1)	807/18,106 (4.5)	0.91	0.83 to 1.01	0.07

*HR; unadjusted.

Abbreviations: CI = confidence interval; HR = hazard ratio; WHI = Women's Health Initiative; y = years.

Table 40. Calcium Evidence Summary

Study Quality	Study design Followup (max)	Supplement and dose Supplement duration	N	Mean age (y)	% Female	CVD incidence	Cancer incidence	Mortality	Harms	Comments
ACS[113,115,185] Fair	RCT 5 years	Calcium 1,000 mg qd 5 years	1,471	74	100	Any: ↔ MI: ↔ Stroke: ↔	NR	↔	↑	Constipation (↑) and hip fractures (↑)
Lappe 2007[109] Fair	RCT 4 years	Calcium 1,400 mg qd 4 years	1,180	67	100	NR	Any: ↔ Lung: ↔ CRC: ↔ Prostate: NA Breast: ↔ Other:	NR	↔	
CPPS[114,116] Fair	RCT 12 years	Calcium 1,200 mg bid 4 years	930	61	28	Any: ↔ MI: NR Stroke: ↔	Any: ↔ Lung: NR CRC: NR Prostate: ↔ Breast: NA Other: NR	↔	↔	
RECORD[103,107] Fair	2x2 factorial RCT 6.2 years	Calcium 1,000 mg qd (alone or in combination with vitamin D$_3$ 800 IU qd) 3.75 years (median) (range, 2 to 5.2 years)	5,292	77	85	Any: ↔* MI: NR Stroke: NR	Any: ↔ Lung: ↔ CRC: ↑ Prostate: ↔ Breast: ↔ Other: ↔	↔	↔	

*CVD mortality only.

Abbreviations: ACS = Auckland Calcium Study; bid = twice daily; CPPS = Calcium Polyp Prevention Study; CRC = colorectal cancer; CVD = cardiovascular disease; max = maximum; MI = myocardial infarction; NA = not applicable; NR = not reported; qd = once daily; RCT = randomized, controlled trial; RECORD = Randomized Evaluation of Calcium or Vitamin D; y = years.

Legend: ↑ (statistically significant increase in risk of outcome from supplementation), ↔ (no statistically significant difference between intervention groups), ↓ (statistically significant decrease in risk of outcome from supplementation).

Table 41. Cardiovascular Disease Incidence and Mortality Among Calcium Studies

Outcome‡	Study	Comparison	Mean followup (y)	Intervention, # of subjects with events (%)	Comparator, # of subjects with events (%)	RR or HR	95% CI	P-value
MI incidence	ACS[113]‡	Calcium vs. placebo	5	31/732 (4.2)	21/739 (2.8)	1.49*	0.86 to 2.57	0.16
Stroke incidence	ACS[113]‡	Calcium vs. placebo	5	34/732 (4.6)	25/739 (3.4)	1.37†	0.83 to 2.28	0.23
	CPPS[114]¶	Calcium vs. placebo	4	12/464 (3)	11/466 (2)	NR	NR	NSD
Any CVD death§	ACS[113]‡	Calcium vs. placebo	5	3/732 (0.4)	6/739 (0.8)	0.51#	0.13 to 2.01	0.51
	RECORD[103]§	Calcium vs. no calcium	6.2	371/2,617 (14.2)	355/2,675 (13.3)	1.07‖	0.92 to 1.24	0.333
Fatal CHD	RECORD[103]	Calcium vs. no calcium	6.2	179/2,617 (6.8)	159/2,675 (5.9)	NR	NR	NR
Fatal stroke	RECORD[103]	Calcium vs. no calcium	6.2	110/2,617 (4.2)	110/2,675 (4.1)	NR	NR	NR

*Incidence rate ratio, 1.67 (95% CI, 0.98 to 2.87); p=0.058.
†Incidence rate ratio, 1.45 (95% CI, 0.88 to 2.49); p=0.15.
‡Adjudicated and verified vascular events (participant report, reported by family member, or from national database of hospital admissions). Angina, other chest pain, and transient ischemic attack were also reported as potential vascular events; however, since they were reported by participants or family only (i.e., not adjudicated or verified), they are not shown here.
§Also reported deaths for other vascular diseases in RECORD.
‖HR.
¶Hospitalizations.
#Mortality rate ratio, 0.51 (95% CI, 0.10 to 2.04); p=0.36.

Abbreviations: ACS = Auckland Calcium Study; CI = confidence interval; CHD = coronary heart disease; CPPS = Calcium Polyp Prevention Study; CVD = cardiovascular disease; HR = hazard ratio; MI = myocardial infarction; NR = not reported; NSD = no significant difference; RECORD = Randomized Evaluation of Calcium or Vitamin D; RR = relative risk; y = years.

Table 42. Cancer Incidence and Mortality Among Calcium Studies

Outcome	Study	Comparison	Mean followup (y)	Intervention, # of subjects with events (%)	Comparator, # of subjects with events (%)	RR or HR	95% CI	P-value
Any cancer incidence	Lappe 2007[109]	Calcium vs. placebo	4	17/445 (3.8)	20/288 (6.9)	0.532	0.27 to 1.03	0.063
	CPPS[116]	Calcium vs. placebo	4	15/464 (3)	21/466 (5)	NR	NR	NSD
	RECORD[103]	Calcium vs. no calcium	6.2	371/2,617 (14.2)	352/2,675 (13.2)	1.06†	0.91 to 1.23	0.485
Breast cancer incidence	Lappe 2007[109]	Calcium vs. placebo	4	6/445 (1.3)	8/288 (2.8)	NR	NR	NR
	RECORD[103]	Calcium vs. no calcium	6.2	41/2,617 (1.6)	39/2,675 (1.5)	NR	NR	NR
Colorectal cancer incidence	Lappe 2007[109]	Calcium vs. placebo	4	0/445 (0)	2/288 (0.7)	NR	NR	NR
	RECORD[103]	Calcium vs. no calcium	6.2	46/2,617 (1.8)	25/2,675 (0.9)	NR	NR	NR
Lung cancer incidence	Lappe 2007[109]	Calcium vs. placebo	4	3/445 (0.7)	3/288 (1.4)	NR	NR	NR
	RECORD[103]	Calcium vs. no calcium	6.2	24/2,617 (0.9)	32/2,675 (1.2)	NR	NR	NR
Prostate cancer incidence	CPPS[114]	Calcium vs. placebo	10.3	33/345 (9.6)	37/327 (11.3)	0.83*	0.52 to 1.32	NR
	RECORD[103]	Calcium vs. no calcium	6.2	12/2,617 (0.5)	17/2,675 (0.6)	NR	NR	NR
Any cancer death	RECORD[103]	Calcium vs. no calcium	6.2	173/2,917 (5.9)	156/2,675 (5.8)	1.13†	0.91 to 1.40	0.249
Breast cancer death	RECORD[103]	Calcium vs. no calcium	6.2	16/2,917 (0.5)	11/2,675 (0.4)	NR	NR	NR
Colorectal cancer death	RECORD[103]	Calcium vs. no calcium	6.2	20/2,917 (0.7)	13/2,675 (0.5)	NR	NR	NR
Lung cancer death	RECORD[103]	Calcium vs. no calcium	6.2	27/2,917 (0.9)	31/2,675 (1.2)	NR	NR	NR
Prostate cancer death	RECORD[103]	Calcium vs. no calcium	6.2	5/2,917 (0.2)	7/2,675 (0.3)	NR	NR	NR

*Rate ratio; also reported between baseline and year 6 (risk ratio, 0.52 [95% CI, 0.28 to 0.98]) and year 2 to year 6 (risk ratio, 0.44 [95% CI, 0.21 to 0.94]).
†HR.

Abbreviations: CI = confidence interval; CPPS = Calcium Polyp Prevention Study; HR = hazard ratio; NR = not reported; NSD = no significant difference; RECORD = Randomized Evaluation of Calcium or Vitamin D; RR = relative risk; y = years

Table 43. All-Cause Mortality Among Calcium Alone vs. Placebo Studies

Study	Comparison	Mean followup (y)	Intervention, # of deaths (%)	Comparator, # of deaths (%)	RR or HR	95% CI	P-value
ACS[113]	Calcium vs. placebo	5	34/732 (4.6)	29/739 (3.9)	1.18	0.73 to 1.92	0.52
CPPS[116]	Calcium vs. placebo	4	25/464 (5)	22/466 (5)	NR	NR	NSD
RECORD[103]*	Calcium vs. no calcium	6.2	862/2,617 (32.9)	855/2,675 (32)	1.03*	0.94 to 1.13	0.460

*HR.

Abbreviations: ACS = Auckland Calcium Study; CI = confidence interval; CPPS = Calcium Polyp Prevention Study; HR = hazard ratio; NR = not reported; NSD = no significant difference; RECORD = Randomized Evaluation of Calcium or Vitamin D; RR = relative risk; y = years.

Table 44. Summary of Evidence of Included Studies

KQ	Supplement	# of studies (k), N randomized (n)†	Design	Major limitations	Consistency	Applicability	Overall quality	Summary of findings
KQ 1 (efficacy)	MVI	k=3, n=27,955	RCT	Only 2 studies examining the efficacy of MVI on cancer and CVD;[49,50] generalizability may be an issue as protective effect seen only in men among healthy subjects; only 1 study included women	Consistent	Moderate-to-high: healthy adult volunteers in France; healthy U.S. male physicians; primary care adult patients in the United States and United Kingdom with cataracts	Good	2 RCTs examining efficacy of MVI on cancer and CVD incidence and mortality,[49,50] minor protective effect against cancer in men but not women; similar pattern for all-cause mortality. Small number of deaths reported in third RCT and likely unreliable.[51]
KQ 2 (harms)	MVI	k=5, n=100,944	RCT (k=4), prospective cohort study (k=1)		Consistent	Moderate-to-high: healthy adult volunteers from France, male physicians and female nurses from the United States; primary care adult patients in the United States and United Kingdom with cataracts; Dutch elderly patients	Good	Increased risk of hip fractures among MVI users compared with nonusers in 1 study (may be due to vitamin A).[53] 4 RCTs reported no difference between groups in the number of hypercarotenemia cases, other side effects, and intercurrent illnesses and respiratory tract infections.[49-52] Mixed results for bleeding.[50]
KQ 3 (efficacy)	Beta-carotene	k=6, n=112,820	RCT	1 trial discontinued early due to increased risk of lung cancer and related deaths;[60] another discontinued due to reported harms from other trials[62]	Consistent	Moderate-to-high: increased risk for lung cancer (smokers and/or asbestos-exposed workers), healthy male physicians or female nurses from the United States; participants with a previous history of BCC and/or SCC	Good	Increased risk of lung cancer incidence and mortality and all-cause mortality among participants at high-risk for lung cancer at baseline (i.e., smokers and/or asbestos-exposed workers).[59,60]
	Vitamin E	k=5, n=120,335	RCT		Consistent	Moderate-to-high: healthy men (general population or physicians) and female nurses; individuals with hypercholesterolemia; male smokers in the United States	Good	No effect on CVD, cancer, or all-cause mortality.

Table 44. Summary of Evidence of Included Studies

KQ	Supplement	# of studies (k), N randomized (n)†	Design	Major limitations	Consistency	Applicability	Overall quality	Summary of findings
	Selenium	k=2, n=36,845	RCT	1 trial discontinued early due to no treatment effect; other study used secondary analyses of CVD and cancer outcomes	Inconsistent	Moderate-to-high: healthy men and men with a previous SCC or BCC from the United States	Good	No effect on CVD or all-cause mortality; however, mixed results for effects on any cancer and site-specific cancers, with 1 small trial finding statistically significant reduced risks[89] and the other finding NSD between selenium alone or when combined with vitamin E.[82]
	Vitamin A	k=2, n=20,611	RCT	Subjects taken out of study during years 4 and 5 due to funding issues in 1 trial; the other trial discontinued early due to increased risk of lung cancer and related deaths associated with beta-carotene supplementation	Consistent	Moderate: participants with a history of actinic keratosis; heavy smokers or asbestos-exposed workers in the United States	Good	Vitamin A appears to have no effect on CVD, cancer, or mortality. Increased risk of lung cancer incidence and mortality and all-cause mortality among participants at high risk for lung cancer at baseline (i.e., smokers and/or asbestos-exposed workers) attributed to beta-carotene component of vitamin A and beta-carotene combination supplement.[60]
	Vitamin C	k=2, n=15,161	RCT	1 study did not report results using its 2x2 factorial design, which may have limited power[79]	Consistent	Moderate: healthy U.S. male physicians and subjects with hypercholesterolemia in Denmark	Fair	No effect on CVD, cancer, or mortality.[79,80]
	Folic acid	k=1, n=1,021	RCT	Secondary analysis of CVD and cancer in a study examining colorectal adenomas	NA	Low: recruited participants with a recent history of colorectal adenomas	Fair	Secondary analysis showed more noncolorectal cancer incident cases in folic acid group than placebo (p=0.02), attributed to higher number of prostate cancers in intervention group. NSD between groups on CVD outcomes.[101]
	Vitamin D	k=2, n=7,978	RCT	Includes a 2x2 factorial study of vitamin D and calcium	Consistent	High: Older adults from United States and United Kingdom	Fair	No effect on CVD, cancer, or mortality.

Table 44. Summary of Evidence of Included Studies

KQ	Supplement	# of studies (k), N randomized (n)†	Design	Major limitations	Consistency	Applicability	Overall quality	Summary of findings
	Calcium	k=4, n=8,873	RCT	Includes a 2x2 factorial study of vitamin D and calcium	Consistent	Moderate: older women from United States, United Kingdom, and New Zealand; results may not be applicable to men or younger age groups	Fair	No effect on CVD, cancer, or mortality; when pooled, 2 trials showed a negative effect on colorectal cancer incidence.[103,109]
	Vitamin D + calcium	k=2, n=37,462	RCT	Women only	Inconsistent	Moderate: older women from United States; results may not be applicable to men or younger age groups	Fair/ Good	1 trial[109] showed a statistically significant decreased risk for developing any cancer while the other trial did not;[108] no effect on CVD or mortality.
	Vitamin B$_1$	k=0	NA	NA	NA	NA	NA	No data
	Vitamin B$_2$	k=0	NA	NA	NA	NA	NA	No data
	Vitamin B$_6$	k=0	NA	NA	NA	NA	NA	No data
	Vitamin B$_{12}$	k=0	NA	NA	NA	NA	NA	No data
	Iron	k=0	NA	NA	NA	NA	NA	No data
	Zinc	k=0	NA	NA	NA	NA	NA	No data
	Magnesium	k=0	NA	NA	NA	NA	NA	No data
	Niacin	k=0	NA	NA	NA	NA	NA	No data
	Calcium + magnesium	k=0	NA	NA	NA	NA	NA	No data
	Folic acid + vitamin B$_{12}$	k=0	NA	NA	NA	NA	NA	No data
	Folic acid + vitamin B$_6$	k=0	NA	NA	NA	NA	NA	No data
KQ 4 (harms)	Beta-carotene	k=6, n=112,820	RCT	1 trial discontinued early due to increased risk of lung cancer and related deaths	Consistent	Moderate-to-high: increased risk for lung cancer (smokers and/or asbestos-exposed workers), healthy male physicians or females from the United States; participants with a previous history of BCC and/or SCC	Good	Aside from paradoxical increase in lung cancer and related deaths among participants at high risk for lung cancer at baseline; no apparent serious harms from beta-carotene supplementation. Yellowing of skin frequently reported.

Table 44. Summary of Evidence of Included Studies

KQ	Supplement	# of studies (k), N randomized (n)†	Design	Major limitations	Consistency	Applicability	Overall quality	Summary of findings
	Vitamin E	k=6, n=120,355	RCT		Consistent	Moderate-to-high: healthy men and women (general population or health care providers); individuals with hypercholesterolemia; male smokers in the United States	Good	Paradoxical effect on hemorrhagic stroke in 1 trial;[80] mixed bleeding outcomes reported in other trials. No other apparent serious harms from vitamin E supplementation.
	Selenium	k=3, n=37,346	RCT	One study discontinued early due to no treatment effects	Inconsistent	Moderate-to-high: healthy men and men with a previous SCC or BCC from the United States; elderly volunteers from the United Kingdom	Good	Mixed dermatological results; 1 study (NPC) found no dermatologic signs of toxicity while the other study (SELECT) found an increased risk of alopecia and mild dermatitis (p<0.01) with selenium supplementation; third trial found no serious harms (U.K. PRECISE).
	Vitamin A	k=5, n=127,998	RCT (k=3), prospective cohort study (k=2)	1 trial discontinued early due to increased risk of lung cancer and related deaths	Consistent	Moderate-to-high: all studies conducted in United States; 2 in all women, 2 in patients with a previous skin condition; 1 in heavy smokers or asbestos-exposed workers	Fair/Good	2 studies in women reported negative impact on bone mass (i.e., increased risk of fractures); no other serious adverse events reported. Paradoxical effect for lung cancer and related death among participants at high risk for lung cancer at baseline (CARET).
	Folic acid	k=1, n=1,021	RCT	Secondary analysis of prostate cancer cases in a study examining colorectal adenomas	NA	Low: recruited participants with a recent history of colorectal adenomas	Fair	Paradoxical effects on prostate cancer incidence; AFPPS did not report on other harms.[101]
	Vitamin D	k=2, n=5,420	RCT	Includes a 2x2 factorial study of vitamin D and calcium	Consistent	Moderate: 1 study in older adults from the United Kingdom; other study in healthy young adults from Australia	Fair	No harms clearly associated with vitamin D supplementation; most attributed to calcium supplementation.

Table 44. Summary of Evidence of Included Studies

KQ	Supplement	# of studies (k), N randomized (n)†	Design	Major limitations	Consistency	Applicability	Overall quality	Summary of findings
	Calcium	k=4, n=8,873	RCT	Includes a 2x2 factorial study of vitamin D and calcium	Consistent	Moderate: older women from United States, United Kingdom, and New Zealand; results may not be applicable to men or younger age groups	Fair	Constipation and other digestive symptoms more frequently reported in calcium groups; renal events as well. Increased risk for hip fractures in calcium group (p=0.013), but not other sites.[113]
	Vitamin D + calcium	k=2, n=37,462	RCT	Women only	Consistent	Moderate: older women from United States; results may not be applicable to men or younger age groups	Fair/ Good	Increased risk of kidney stones reported in 1 trial;[108] NSD between combination and placebo group on other harms.
	Iron	k=0	NA	NA	NA	NA	NA	No data

†N randomized reported for entire study population.

Abbreviations: AFPPS = Aspirin/Folate Polyp Prevention Study; BCC = basal cell carcinoma; CARET = Carotene and Retinol Efficacy Trial; CVD = cardiovascular disease; KQ = key question; MVI = multivitamin; NA = not applicable; NPC = Nutritional Prevention of Cancer; NSD = no significant difference; RCT = randomized, controlled trial; SCC = squamous cell carcinoma; SELECT = Selenium and Vitamin E Cancer Prevention Trial; U.K. PRECISE = U.K. Prevention of Cancer by Intervention with Selenium.

Appendix A. Dietary Reference Intakes

Vitamin or mineral	Other names	Group	Age (years)*	RDA	UL
Vitamin A (mcg/d)	Vitamin A, retinol, retinal	Males	9–13	600	1700
			14–18	900	2800
			≥19	900	3000
		Females	9–13	600	1700
			14–18	700	2800
			≥19	700	3000
Vitamin B_1 (mg/d)	Thiamine, thiamin, aneurine	Males	9–13	0.9	ND
			≥14	1.2	ND
		Females	9–13	0.9	ND
			14–18	1.0	ND
			≥19	1.1	ND
Vitamin B_2 (mg/d)	Riboflavin	Males	9–13	0.9	ND
			≥14	1.3	ND
		Females	9–13	0.9	ND
			14–18	1.0	ND
			≥19	1.1	ND
Vitamin B_6 (mg/d)	None	Males	9–13	1.0	60
			14–18	1.3	80
			19–50	1.3	100
			≥51	1.7	100
		Females	9–13	1.0	60
			14–18	1.2	80
			19–50	1.3	100
			≥51	1.5	100
Vitamin B_{12} (mcg/d)	Cobalamin	Males	9–13	1.8	ND
			≥14	2.4	ND
		Females	9–13	1.8	ND
			≥14	2.4	ND
Vitamin C (mg/d)	L-ascorbic acid, ascorbate, dehydroascorbic acid (DHA)	Males	9–13	45	1200
			14–18	75	1800
			≥19	90	2000
		Females	4–8	75	1200
			9–18	65	1800
			≥19	75	2000
Vitamin D (mcg/d)	Calciferol	Males	9–70	15	100
			≥71	20	100
		Females	9–70	15	100
			≥71	20	100
Vitamin E (mg/d)	alpha-tocopherol	Males	9–13	11	600
			14–18	15	800
			≥19	15	1000
		Females	9–13	11	600
			14–18	15	800
			≥19	15	1000
Calcium (mg/d)	Calcium carbonate, calcium gluconate, calcium citrate	Males	9–13	1300	3000
			19–30	1000	2500
			51–70	1000	2000
			≥71	1200	2000
		Females	9–13	1300	3000
			19–30	1000	2500
			≥51	1200	2000
Folic acid (mcg/d)	Vitamin M, vitamin B_9, vitamin B_c, folacin, pteroyl-L-glutamic acid, pteroyl-L-glutamate, pteroylmonoglutamic acid, folate	Males	9–13	300	600
			14–18	400	800
			≥19	400	1000
		Females	9–13	300	600
			14–18	400	800
			≥19	400	1000

Appendix A. Dietary Reference Intakes

Vitamin or mineral	Other names	Group	Age (years)*	RDA	UL
Iron (mg/d)	None	Males	9–13	8	40
			14–18	11	45
			≥19	8	45
		Females	9–13	8	40
			14–18	15	45
			19–30	18	45
			31–50	15	45
			≥51	8	45
Magnesium (mg/d)	Magnesia, magnesia carbonica, magnesia muriatica, magnesium gluconate, milk of magnesia	Males	9–13	240	350
			14–18	410	350
			19–30	400	350
			≥31	420	350
		Females	9–13	240	350
			14–18	360	350
			19–30	310	350
			≥31	320	350
Niacin (mg/d)	Vitamin B_3, nicotinic acid, vitamin PP	Males	9–13	12	20
			14–18	16	30
			≥19	16	35
		Females	9–13	12	20
			14–18	14	30
			≥19	14	35
Selenium (mcg/d)	High-selenium yeast, selenized yeast, chelated selenium	Males	9–13	40	280
			≥14	55	400
		Females	9–13	40	280
			≥14	55	400
Zinc (mg/d)	Zinc acetate	Males	9–13	8	23
			14–18	11	34
			≥19	11	40
		Females	9–13	8	23
			14–18	9	34
			≥19	8	40

*Data for children younger than age 9 years are available in original source documents.

Abbreviations: ND = not determinable; RDA = recommended dietary allowance; UL = upper intake level.

Note: Beta-carotene does not have a dietary reference intake.

Appendix B. Literature Search Strategies

Database: **Ovid MEDLINE**(R) without Revisions <1996 to April Week 4 2012>, Ovid MEDLINE(R) Daily Update <January 29, 2013>

---

1. Calcium, dietary/
2. dietary calcium.ti,ab.
3. calcium supplement*.ti,ab.
4. folic acid/
5. folic acid.ti,ab.
6. folate.ti,ab.
7. Thiamine/
8. Thiamine.ti,ab.
9. Thiamin.ti,ab.
10. Thiamine Monophosphate/
11. Thiamine Pyrophosphate/
12. Thiamine Triphosphate/
13. Vitamin B 1.ti,ab.
14. Vitamin B1.ti,ab.
15. Aneurin.ti,ab.
16. Riboflavin/
17. Riboflavin.ti,ab.
18. Vitamin B 2.ti,ab.
19. Vitamin B2.ti,ab.
20. Vitamin B 6/
21. Vitamin B 6.ti,ab.
22. Vitamin B6.ti,ab.
23. Pyridoxine/
24. Pyridoxine.ti,ab.
25. Vitamin B 12/
26. Vitamin B 12.ti,ab.
27. Vitamin B12.ti,ab.
28. Cobamides/
29. Hydroxocobalamin/
30. Cobalamin.ti,ab.
31. Cyanocobalamin.ti,ab.
32. Cobamides.ti,ab.
33. Hydroxocobalamin.ti,ab.
34. Vitamin D/
35. Vitamin D.ti,ab.
36. Cholecalciferol/
37. Cholecalciferol.ti,ab.
38. Dihydroxycholecalciferols/
39. Dihydroxycholecalciferol*.ti,ab.
40. Calcitriol/
41. Calcitriol.ti,ab.
42. Ergocalciferols/
43. Ergocalciferol*.ti,ab.

Appendix B. Literature Search Strategies

44	Vitamin E/
45	Vitamin E.ti,ab.
46	Tocopherols/
47	Tocopherol*.ti,ab.
48	Tocotrienols/
49	Tocotrienol*.ti,ab.
50	Ascorbic acid/
51	Ascorbic acid.ti,ab.
52	Vitamin C.ti,ab.
53	ascorbate.ti,ab.
54	Vitamin A/
55	Vitamin A.ti,ab.
56	beta carotene/
57	beta carotene.ti,ab.
58	Retinol.ti,ab.
59	iron, dietary/
60	(iron adj5 dietary).ti,ab.
61	(iron adj5 supplement*).ti,ab.
62	zinc/
63	(zinc adj5 dietary).ti,ab.
64	(zinc adj5 supplement*).ti,ab.
65	Magnesium/
66	Magnesium Compounds/
67	(magnesium adj5 dietary).ti,ab.
68	(magnesium adj5 supplement*).ti,ab.
69	Niacin/
70	Niacin.ti,ab.
71	Nicotinic acids/
72	Nicotinic acid*.ti,ab.
73	Selenium/
74	Selenium compounds/
75	Selenium.ti,ab.
76	Vitamins/
77	Minerals/
78	(Vitamin* adj5 dietary).ti,ab.
79	(Vitamin* adj5 supplement*).ti,ab.
80	(mineral* adj5 dietary).ti,ab.
81	(mineral* adj5 supplement*).ti,ab.
82	Multivitamin*.ti,ab.
83	multimineral*.ti,ab.
84	or/1-83
85	Cardiovascular Diseases/
86	Heart Diseases/
87	cardiovascular disease*.ti,ab.
88	heart disease*.ti,ab.
89	exp Arrhythmias, Cardiac/

Appendix B. Literature Search Strategies

90 exp Cardiomyopathies/
91 exp Heart Arrest/
92 exp Heart Failure/
93 exp Myocardial Ischemia/
94 exp Ventricular Dysfunction/
95 myocardial infarction.ti,ab.
96 Heart arrest.ti,ab.
97 myocardial isch?emia.ti,ab.
98 Coronary artery disease.ti,ab.
99 heart attack*.ti,ab.
100 Isch?emic heart disease.ti,ab.
101 Vascular Diseases/
102 exp Aneurysm/
103 exp Arterial Occlusive Diseases/
104 Cerebrovascular Disorders/
105 exp Carotid Artery Diseases/
106 exp Stroke/
107 exp Diabetic Angiopathies/
108 exp Hypertension/
109 Peripheral Vascular Diseases/
110 Peripheral Arterial Disease/
111 Prehypertension/
112 Stroke.ti,ab.
113 Hypertension.ti,ab.
114 Cerebrovascular disease*.ti,ab.
115 Cerebrovascular disorder*.ti,ab.
116 Carotid artery disease*.ti,ab.
117 exp Hyperlipidemias/
118 Hyperlipid?emia*.ti,ab.
119 Hypercholesterol?emia*.ti,ab.
120 High cholesterol.ti,ab.
121 Elevated cholesterol.ti,ab.
122 Neoplasms/
123 exp Abdominal Neoplasms/
124 exp Bone Neoplasms/
125 exp Breast Neoplasms/
126 exp Digestive System Neoplasms/
127 exp Endocrine Gland Neoplasms/
128 exp Eye Neoplasms/
129 exp "Head and Neck Neoplasms"/
130 exp Hematologic Neoplasms/
131 exp Nervous System Neoplasms/
132 exp Pelvic Neoplasms/
133 exp Skin Neoplasms/
134 exp Soft Tissue Neoplasms/
135 Splenic Neoplasms/

Appendix B. Literature Search Strategies

136	exp Thoracic Neoplasms/
137	exp Urogenital Neoplasms/
138	exp Intestinal Polyps/
139	lung cancer.ti,ab.
140	lung neoplas*.ti,ab.
141	breast cancer.ti,ab.
142	Breast neoplas*.ti,ab.
143	colorectal cancer.ti,ab.
144	Colorectal neoplas*.ti,ab.
145	prostate cancer.ti,ab.
146	Prostatic neoplas*.ti,ab.
147	gastric cancer.ti,ab.
148	stomach cancer.ti,ab.
149	Stomach neoplas*.ti,ab.
150	Abdominal neoplas*.ti,ab.
151	colorectal polyps.ti,ab.
152	Colon* polyps.ti,ab.
153	adenomas.ti,ab.
154	or/85-153
155	84 and 154
156	Randomized controlled trial.pt.
157	controlled clinical trial.pt.
158	Meta analysis.pt.
159	Random allocation/
160	double-blind method/
161	single-blind method/
162	Random*.ti,ab.
163	(control* adj3 trial*).ti,ab.
164	placebo*.ti,ab.
165	controlled clinical trials as topic/
166	randomized controlled trials as topic/
167	meta analysis as topic/
168	systematic review*.ti,ab.
169	systematic evidence review*.ti,ab.
170	meta analy*.ti,ab.
171	metaanaly*.ti,ab.
172	or/156-171
173	155 and 172
174	limit 173 to animals
175	limit 173 to humans
176	174 not 175
177	173 not 176
178	limit 177 to english language
179	limit 178 to yr="2005 -Current"
180	Calcium, dietary/
181	dietary calcium.ti,ab.

Appendix B. Literature Search Strategies

182	calcium supplement*.ti,ab.
183	folic acid/
184	folic acid.ti,ab.
185	folate.ti,ab.
186	Vitamin D/
187	Vitamin D.ti,ab.
188	Cholecalciferol/
189	Cholecalciferol.ti,ab.
190	Dihydroxycholecalciferols/
191	Dihydroxycholecalciferol*.ti,ab.
192	Calcitriol/
193	Calcitriol.ti,ab.
194	Ergocalciferols/
195	Ergocalciferol*.ti,ab.
196	Vitamin E/
197	Vitamin E.ti,ab.
198	Tocopherols/
199	Tocopherol*.ti,ab.
200	Tocotrienols/
201	Tocotrienol*.ti,ab.
202	Vitamin A/
203	Vitamin A.ti,ab.
204	beta carotene/
205	beta carotene.ti,ab.
206	Retinol.ti,ab.
207	iron, dietary/
208	(iron adj5 dietary).ti,ab.
209	(iron adj5 supplement*).ti,ab.
210	Selenium/
211	Selenium compounds/
212	Selenium.ti,ab.
213	Vitamins/
214	Minerals/
215	(Vitamin* adj5 dietary).ti,ab.
216	(Vitamin* adj5 supplement*).ti,ab.
217	(mineral* adj5 dietary).ti,ab.
218	(mineral* adj5 supplement*).ti,ab.
219	Multivitamin*.ti,ab.
220	multimineral*.ti,ab.
221	or/180-220
222	safety/
223	safety.ti,ab.
224	adverse event*.ti,ab.
225	adverse effects.fs.
226	adverse effect*.ti,ab.
227	side effect*.ti,ab.

Appendix B. Literature Search Strategies

228	product surveillance, postmarketing/
229	Adverse reaction*.ti,ab.
230	Adverse drug reaction*.ti,ab.
231	drug toxicity/
232	drug toxicity.ti,ab.
233	Harm*.ti,ab.
234	or/222-233
235	221 and 234
236	case-control studies/
237	retrospective studies/
238	cohort studies/
239	longitudinal studies/
240	follow-up studies/
241	prospective studies/
242	Cross-Sectional Studies/
243	cohort.ti,ab.
244	longitudinal.ti,ab.
245	follow up.ti,ab.
246	followup.ti,ab.
247	prospective*.ti,ab.
248	retrospective*.ti,ab.
249	comparison group*.ti,ab.
250	control group*.ti,ab.
251	observational.ti,ab.
252	nonrandom*.ti,ab.
253	database*.ti,ab.
254	population*.ti,ab.
255	cross sectional.ti,ab.
256	or/236-255
257	235 and 256
258	limit 257 to humans
259	limit 257 to animals
260	259 not 258
261	257 not 260
262	limit 261 to english language
263	limit 262 to yr="2005 -Current"
264	179 or 263

Database: **Cochrane Database of Systematic Reviews, CENTRAL and DARE**
Search Strategy:

#1	"cardiovascular disease":ti,ab,kw, from 2005 to 2013
#2	"cardiovascular diseases":ti,ab,kw, from 2005 to 2013
#3	"heart disease":ti,ab,kw, from 2005 to 2013
#4	"heart diseases":ti,ab,kw , from 2005 to 2013
#5	Arrhythmia*:ti,ab,kw, from 2005 to 2013

Appendix B. Literature Search Strategies

#6   Cardiomyopath*:ti,ab,kw, from 2005 to 2013
#7   "Heart Arrest":ti,ab,kw, from 2005 to 2013
#8   "Heart Failure":ti,ab,kw, from 2005 to 2013
#9   "Myocardial Ischemia":ti,ab,kw, from 2005 to 2013
#10 "Ventricular Dysfunction":ti,ab,kw, from 2005 to 2013
#11 "myocardial infarction":ti,ab,kw, from 2005 to 2013
#12 "Coronary artery disease":ti,ab,kw, from 2005 to 2013
#13 "heart attack":ti,ab,kw, from 2005 to 2013
#14 "heart attacks":ti,ab,kw, from 2005 to 2013
#15 "Ischemic heart disease":ti,ab,kw, from 2005 to 2013
#16 "Vascular Diseases":ti,ab,kw, from 2005 to 2013
#17 "Vascular Disease":ti,ab,kw, from 2005 to 2013
#18 Aneurysm*:ti,ab,kw, from 2005 to 2013
#19 "Arterial Occlusive":ti,ab,kw, from 2005 to 2013
#20 Cerebrovascular:ti,ab,kw, from 2005 to 2013
#21 "Carotid Artery":ti,ab,kw, from 2005 to 2013
#22 stroke:ti,ab,kw, from 2005 to 2013
#23 "Diabetic Angiopathies":ti,ab,kw, from 2005 to 2013
#24 "Diabetic Angiopathy":ti,ab,kw, from 2005 to 2012
#25 Hypertension:ti,ab,kw, from 2005 to 2013
#26 "Peripheral Vascular":ti,ab,kw, from 2005 to 2013
#27 "Peripheral Arterial":ti,ab,kw, from 2005 to 2013
#28 Prehypertension:ti,ab,kw, from 2005 to 2013
#29 Hyperlipidemia*:ti,ab,kw, from 2005 to 2013
#30 Hypercholesterolemia*:ti,ab,kw, from 2005 to 2013
#31 "High cholesterol":ti,ab,kw, from 2005 to 2013
#32 "elevated cholesterol":ti,ab,kw, from 2005 to 2013
#33 "Abdominal Neoplasms":ti,ab,kw, from 2005 to 2013
#34 "Bone Neoplasms":ti,ab,kw, from 2005 to 2013
#35 "Breast Neoplasms":ti,ab,kw, from 2005 to 2013
#36 Digestive near/2 Neoplasms:ti,ab,kw, from 2005 to 2013
#37 endocrine near/2 Neoplasms:ti,ab,kw, from 2005 to 2013
#38 "Eye Neoplasms":ti,ab,kw, from 2005 to 2013
#39 Head near/3 Neoplasms:ti,ab,kw, from 2005 to 2013
#40 neck near/3 Neoplasms:ti,ab,kw, from 2005 to 2013
#41 "Hematologic Neoplasms":ti,ab,kw, from 2005 to 2013
#42 "Nervous System Neoplasms":ti,ab,kw, from 2005 to 2013
#43 "Pelvic Neoplasms":ti,ab,kw, from 2005 to 2013
#44 "Skin Neoplasms":ti,ab,kw, from 2005 to 2013
#45 "Soft Tissue Neoplasms":ti,ab,kw, from 2005 to 2013
#46 "Splenic Neoplasms":ti,ab,kw, from 2005 to 2013
#47 "Thoracic Neoplasms":ti,ab,kw, from 2005 to 2013
#48 "Urogenital Neoplasms":ti,ab,kw, from 2005 to 2013
#49 "Intestinal Polyps":ti,ab,kw, from 2005 to 2013
#50 "lung cancer":ti,ab,kw, from 2005 to 2013
#51 "breast cancer":ti,ab,kw, from 2005 to 2013

Appendix B. Literature Search Strategies

#52 "colorectal cancer":ti,ab,kw, from 2005 to 2013
#53 "colon cancer":ti,ab,kw, from 2005 to 2013
#54 "prostate cancer":ti,ab,kw, from 2005 to 2013
#55 "gastric cancer":ti,ab,kw, from 2005 to 2013
#56 "stomach cancer":ti,ab,kw, from 2005 to 2013
#57 "colorectal polyps":ti,ab,kw, from 2005 to 2013
#58 "Colon polyps":ti,ab,kw, from 2005 to 2013
#59 "Colonic polyps":ti,ab,kw, from 2005 to 2013
#60 adenomas:ti,ab,kw, from 2005 to 2013
#61 (#1 OR #2 OR #3 OR #4 OR #5 OR #6 OR #7 OR #8 OR #9 OR #10 OR #11 OR #12 OR #13 OR #14 OR #15 OR #16 OR #17 OR #18 OR #19 OR #20 OR #21 OR #22 OR #23 OR #24 OR #25 OR #26 OR #27 OR #28 OR #29 OR #30 OR #31 OR #32 OR #33 OR #34 OR #35 OR #36 OR #37 OR #38 OR #39 OR #40 OR #41 OR #42 OR #43 OR #44 OR #45 OR #46 OR #47 OR #48 OR #49 OR #50 OR #51 OR #52 OR #53 OR #54 OR #55 OR #56 OR #57 OR #58 OR #59 OR #60), from 2005 to 2013
#62 (Calcium near/2 dietary):ti,ab,kw
#63 (calcium next supplement*):ti,ab,kw
#64 "folic acid":ti,ab,kw
#65 folate:ti,ab,kw
#66 Thiamine:ti,ab,kw
#67 thiamin:ti,ab,kw
#68 "Vitamin B 1":ti,ab,kw
#69 "vitamin b1":ti,ab,kw
#70 Aneurin:ti,ab,kw
#71 Riboflavin:ti,ab,kw
#72 "Vitamin B 2":ti,ab,kw
#73 "Vitamin B2":ti,ab,kw
#74 "Vitamin B 6":ti,ab,kw
#75 "Vitamin B6":ti,ab,kw
#76 Pyridoxine:ti,ab,kw
#77 "Vitamin B 12":ti,ab,kw
#78 "Vitamin B12":ti,ab,kw
#79 Cobamides:ti,ab,kw
#80 Hydroxocobalamin:ti,ab,kw
#81 Cobalamin:ti,ab,kw
#82 Cyanocobalamin:ti,ab,kw
#83 "Vitamin D":ti,ab,kw
#84 Cholecalciferol:ti,ab,kw
#85 Dihydroxycholecalciferol*:ti,ab,kw
#86 Calcitriol:ti,ab,kw
#87 Ergocalciferol*:ti,ab,kw
#88 "Vitamin E":ti,ab,kw
#89 Tocopherol*:ti,ab,kw
#90 Tocotrienol*:ti,ab,kw
#91 "Ascorbic acid":ti,ab,kw
#92 "Vitamin C":ti,ab,kw

Appendix B. Literature Search Strategies

#93 ascorbate:ti,ab,kw
#94 "Vitamin A":ti,ab,kw
#95 "beta carotene":ti,ab,kw
#96 Retinol:ti,ab,kw
#97 (iron near/2 dietary):ti,ab,kw
#98 (iron next supplement*):ti,ab,kw
#99 zinc:ti,ab,kw
#100 Magnesium:ti,ab,kw
#101 Niacin:ti,ab,kw
#102 (Nicotinic near/2 acid*):ti,ab,kw
#103 Selenium:ti,ab,kw
#104 (vitamin* near/2 dietary):ti,ab,kw
#105 (vitamin* near/2 supplement*):ti,ab,kw
#106 Multivitamin*:ti,ab,kw
#107 multimineral*:ti,ab,kw
#108 (#62 OR #63 OR #64 OR #65 OR #66 OR #67 OR #68 OR #69 OR #70 OR #71 OR #72 OR #73 OR #74 OR #75 OR #76 OR #77 OR #78 OR #79 OR #80 OR #81 OR #82 OR #83 OR #84 OR #85 OR #86 OR #87 OR #88 OR #89 OR #90 OR #91 OR #92 OR #93 OR #94 OR #95 OR #96 OR #97 OR #98 OR #99 OR #100 OR #101 OR #102 OR #103 OR #104 OR #105 OR #106 OR #107)
#109 (#61 AND #108), from 2005 to 2013

Database: **EMBASE**
Search Strategy:

'calcium intake':de OR 'folic acid':de OR 'thiamine':de OR 'thiamine phosphate':de OR 'thiamine triphosphate':de OR 'riboflavin':de OR 'pyridoxine':de OR 'cobamamide':de OR 'cyanocobalamin':de OR 'hydroxocobalamin':de OR 'vitamin d':de AND r AND 'colecalciferol':de OR 'dihydroxycolecalciferol':de OR 'calcitriol':de OR 'ergocalciferol':de OR 'alpha tocopherol':de OR 'tocopherol':de OR 'alpha tocotrienol':de OR 'ascorbic acid':de OR 'beta carotene':de OR 'retinol':de OR 'iron intake':de OR 'zinc':de OR 'magnesium':de OR 'magnesium derivative':de OR 'nicotinic acid':de OR 'selenium':de OR 'selenium derivative':de OR 'vitamin':de OR 'multivitamin':de OR 'ferrous sulfate plus multivitamin':de OR 'mineral':de AND ('cardiovascular disease':de OR 'heart disease':de OR 'heart arrhythmia'/exp OR 'cardiomyopathy'/exp OR 'heart failure'/exp OR 'heart muscle ischemia':de OR 'heart infarction'/exp OR 'coronary artery disease':de OR 'vascular disease':de OR 'aneurysm'/exp OR 'peripheral occlusive artery disease'/exp OR 'cerebrovascular disease':de OR 'carotid artery disease'/exp OR 'stroke':de OR 'diabetic angiopathy'/exp OR 'hypertension'/exp OR 'peripheral vascular disease':de OR 'peripheral occlusive artery disease':de OR 'hyperlipidemia'/exp OR 'neoplasm':de OR 'neoplasms subdivided by anatomical site'/exp OR 'intestine polyp'/exp OR 'adenomatous polyp':de) AND ('randomized controlled trial':de OR 'randomized controlled trial (topic)':de OR 'controlled clinical trial':de OR 'controlled clinical trial (topic)':de OR 'meta analysis':de OR 'meta analysis (topic)':de OR 'randomization':de OR 'double blind procedure':de OR 'single blind procedure':de OR 'placebo':de OR 'systematic review':de OR 'systematic review (topic)':de) AND [humans]/lim AND [english]/lim AND [embase]/lim AND [2005-2013]/py

Appendix B. Literature Search Strategies

'calcium intake':de OR 'folic acid':de OR 'vitamin d':de OR 'colecalciferol':de OR 'dihydroxycolecalciferol':de OR 'calcitriol':de OR 'ergocalciferol':de OR 'alpha tocopherol':de OR 'tocopherol':de OR 'alpha tocotrienol':de OR 'beta carotene':de OR 'retinol':de OR 'iron intake':de OR 'selenium':de OR 'selenium derivative':de OR 'vitamin':de OR 'multivitamin':de OR 'ferrous sulfate plus multivitamin':de OR 'mineral':de AND ('safety':de OR 'adverse drug reaction'/exp OR 'postmarketing surveillance':de OR 'drug surveillance program':de OR 'drug toxicity':de) AND ('case control study':de OR 'population based case control study':de OR 'retrospective study':de OR 'cohort analysis':de OR 'longitudinal study':de OR 'follow up':de OR 'prospective study':de OR 'cross-sectional study':de OR 'control group':de OR 'observational study':de) AND [humans]/lim AND [english]/lim AND [embase]/lim AND [2005-2013]/py

Appendix B Figure 1. Literature Flow Diagram

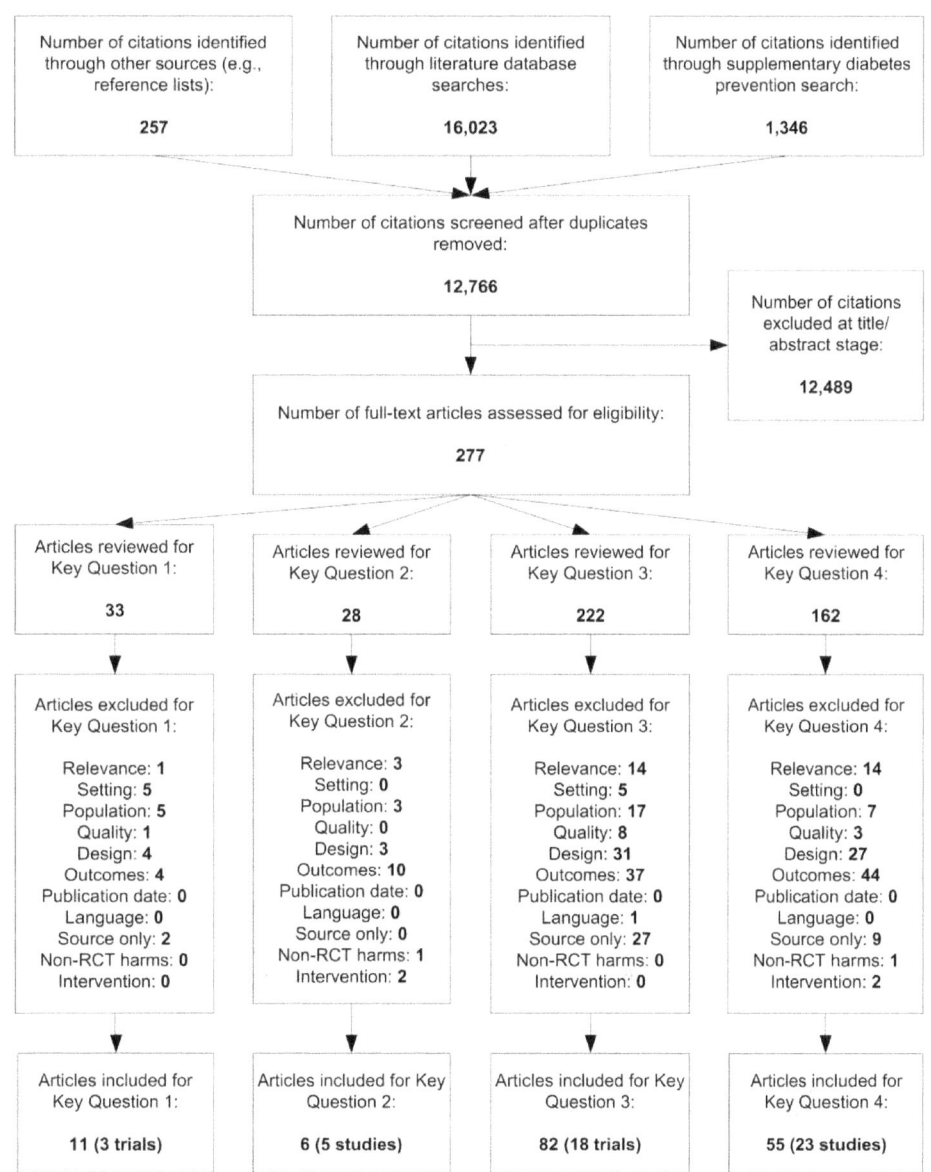

Abbreviation: RCT = randomized, controlled trial.

Appendix B Table 1. Inclusion and Exclusion Criteria

Category	Inclusion	Exclusion
Populations	**Efficacy (KQs 1, 3):** Community-dwelling adults (age ≥18 years) without chronic disease and without nutritional deficiencies. **Harms (KQs 2, 4):** Community-dwelling adults and children (any age) without chronic disease.	Nonhuman populations; populations that only/exclusively included pregnant women, infants, individuals with a particular chronic disease, individuals receiving supplements as treatment for chronic disease (e.g., cancer, cardiovascular disease, HIV, end-stage renal disease, chronic kidney disease, tuberculosis), dialysis patients, individuals with clinical nutritional deficiencies, institutionalized individuals, organ transplant recipients, or hospitalized individuals.
Disease/ condition	**KQs 1, 3:** Primary prevention of cancer and cardiovascular disease; i.e., oncologic (breast, colorectal, lung, prostate, and gastric cancer; any other malignancy), cardiovascular (myocardial infarction, stroke).	Secondary and tertiary prevention or nutritional deficiencies.
Interventions	**KQs 1, 2:** Multivitamins defined as three or more vitamins and/or minerals without herbs, hormones, or drugs, each at a dose less than the UL as determined by the Food and Nutrition Board. **KQ 3:** Single nutrients and functionally related pairs each at a dose less than the UL as determined by the Food and Nutrition Board (i.e., calcium; folic acid; vitamins B_1, B_2, B_6, B_{12}, D, E, C, A; iron; zinc; magnesium; niacin; selenium; beta-carotene; calcium/vitamin D; calcium/magnesium; folic acid/vitamin B_{12}; and folic acid/vitamin B_6). **KQ 4:** Single nutrients and functionally related pairs each at a dose less than the UL as determined by the Food and Nutrition Board (i.e., calcium; folic acid; vitamins D, E, A; iron; selenium; beta-carotene; and calcium/vitamin D).	Did not address the use of supplements separately from dietary intake.
Comparisons	Not specified.	Not specified.
Outcomes	**Efficacy (KQs 1, 3):** Primary or secondary endpoint of disease or condition including mortality, will also accept study-specified surrogate outcomes (but must also report disease outcome). **Harms (KQs 2, 4):** Any harms (e.g., self-reported symptoms/adverse events, objective measurements such as blood or urine tests).	**Efficacy (KQs 1, 3):** Did not report disease or condition as primary or secondary outcome; precancerous outcomes (e.g., adenomas) without overt cancer outcomes. **Harms (KQs 2, 4):** Not specified.
Study designs	**Efficacy (KQs 1, 3):** Systematic reviews, RCTs. **Harms (KQs 2, 4):** RCTs or observational studies (including case reports and case series), postmarket surveillance data.	**Efficacy (KQs 1, 3):** Narrative reviews, nonrandomized studies. **Harms (KQs 2, 4):** Editorial, commentary, letter.

Abbreviations: KQ = key question; RCT = randomized, controlled trial; UL = upper intake level.

Appendix B Table 2. Quality Assessment Criteria

Design	U.S. Preventive Services Task Force quality rating criteria[187]	National Institute for Health and Clinical Excellence methodology checklists[46]
Systematic reviews and meta-analyses	<ul><li>Comprehensiveness of sources considered/search strategy used</li><li>Standard appraisal of included studies</li><li>Validity of conclusions</li><li>Recency and relevance are especially important for systematic reviews</li></ul>	<ul><li>Study addresses an appropriate and clearly focused question</li><li>Description of the methodology used is included</li><li>Literature search is sufficiently rigorous to identify all the relevant studies</li><li>Study quality is assessed and taken into account</li><li>There are enough similarities between the studies selected to make combining them reasonable</li></ul>
Case-control studies	<ul><li>Accurate ascertainment of cases</li><li>Nonbiased selection of cases/controls with exclusion criteria applied equally to both</li><li>Response rate</li><li>Diagnostic testing procedures applied equally to each group</li><li>Measurement of exposure accurate and applied equally to each group</li><li>Appropriate attention to potential confounding variables</li></ul>	<ul><li>Study addresses an appropriate and clearly focused question</li><li>Cases and controls are taken from comparable populations</li><li>Same exclusion criteria are used for both cases and controls</li><li>Reports percentage of each group (cases and controls) who participated in the study</li><li>Comparison is made between participants and nonparticipants to establish their similarities or differences</li><li>Cases are clearly defined and differentiated from controls</li><li>Controls are clearly established from noncases</li><li>Measures have been taken to prevent knowledge of primary exposure influencing case ascertainment</li><li>Exposure status is measured in a standard, valid, and reliable way</li><li>Main potential confounders are identified and taken into account in the design and analysis</li><li>Confidence intervals are provided</li></ul>
Randomized, controlled trials	<ul><li>Initial assembly of comparable groups employs adequate randomization, including first concealment and whether potential confounders were distributed equally among groups</li><li>Maintenance of comparable groups (includes attrition, crossovers, adherence, contamination)</li><li>Important differential loss to followup or overall high loss to followup</li><li>Measurements are equal, reliable, and valid (includes masking of outcome assessment)</li><li>Clear definition of the interventions</li><li>All important outcomes considered</li></ul>	<ul><li>Study addresses an appropriate and clearly focused question</li><li>Assignment of subjects to treatment groups is randomized</li><li>Adequate concealment method is used</li><li>Subjects and investigators are kept "blind" about treatment allocation</li><li>Treatment and control groups are similar at the start of the trial</li><li>Only difference between groups is the treatment under investigation</li><li>All relevant outcomes are measured in a standard, valid, and reliable way</li><li>Reports percentage of individuals or clusters recruited into each treatment arm of the study who dropped out before the study was completed</li><li>All subjects are analyzed in the groups to which they were randomly allocated (often referred to as intention-to-treat analysis)</li><li>When the study is carried out at more than one site, results are comparable for all sites</li></ul>

Appendix B Table 2. Quality Assessment Criteria

Design	U.S. Preventive Services Task Force quality rating criteria[187]	National Institute for Health and Clinical Excellence methodology checklists[45]
Cohort studies	<ul><li>Initial assembly of comparable groups employs consideration of potential confounders with either restriction or measurement for adjustment in the analysis; consideration of inception cohorts</li><li>Maintenance of comparable groups (includes attrition, crossovers, adherence, contamination)</li><li>Important differential loss to followup or overall high loss to followup</li><li>Measurements are equal, reliable, and valid (includes masking of outcome assessment)</li><li>Clear definition of the interventions</li><li>All important outcomes considered</li></ul>	<ul><li>Study addresses an appropriate and clearly focused question</li><li>Two groups being studied are selected from source populations that are comparable in all respects other than the factor under investigation</li><li>Study indicates how many of the people asked to take part did so, in each of the groups being studied</li><li>Likelihood that some eligible subjects might have the outcome at the time of enrollment is assessed and taken into account in the analysis</li><li>Reports percentage of individuals or clusters recruited into each arm of the study who dropped out before the study was completed</li><li>Comparison is made between full participants and those lost to followup, by exposure status</li><li>Outcomes are clearly defined</li><li>Assessment of outcome is made blind to exposure status</li><li>When blinding was not possible, there is some recognition that knowledge of exposure status could have influenced the assessment of outcome</li><li>Measure of assessment of exposure is reliable</li><li>Evidence from other sources is used to demonstrate that the method of outcome assessment is valid and reliable</li><li>Exposure level or prognostic factor is assessed more than once</li><li>Main potential confounders are identified and taken into account in the design and analysis</li><li>Confidence intervals are provided</li></ul>
Diagnostic accuracy studies	<ul><li>Screening test relevant, available for primary care, and adequately described</li><li>Study uses a credible reference standard, performed regardless of test results</li><li>Reference standard interpreted independently of screening test</li><li>Handles indeterminate result in a reasonable manner</li><li>Spectrum of patients included in study</li><li>Sample size</li><li>Administration of reliable screening test</li></ul>	<ul><li>Nature of the test being studied is clearly specified</li><li>Test is compared with an appropriate gold standard</li><li>Where no gold standard exists, a validated reference standard is used as a comparator</li><li>Patients for testing are selected either as a consecutive series or randomly, from a clearly defined study population</li><li>Test and gold standard are measured independently (blind) of each other</li><li>Test and gold standard are applied as close together in time as possible</li><li>Results are reported for all patients that are entered into the study</li><li>A prediagnosis is made and reported</li></ul>

Appendix C. Ongoing or Recently Completed Studies

Study	Design	Aim	Location	Number of participants	Intervention description	Relevant outcomes	2013 status
Adjei 2012[188]	Open-label	Determine side effects and best dose of calcitriol in preventing lung cancer in current and former smokers at high risk for lung cancer	United States	NR	Oral vitamin D every 2 weeks	Adverse effects, toxicities	Estimated completion, December 2015
Camargo, 2011[189]	RCT	Determine the effect of vitamin D supplementation on cardiovascular disease event rates	New Zealand	5,100	Vitamin D_3 200,000 IU at baseline; 100,000 IU monthly	Cardiovascular disease	Estimated completion, 2017
Goossens 2012 (Selenium and Bladder Cancer Trial)[190]	RCT	Determine the effect of selenium supplementation on bladder cancer recurrence	Belgium	900	Selenium 200 mcg qd	Serious adverse events	Estimated completion, October 2014
Lance 2011 (Selenium and Vitamin E Cancer Prevention Trial)[191]	RCT	Determine the effect of vitamin E and/or selenium on colorectal polyps in men enrolled in the SELECT trial	United States	NR	Selenium ± vitamin E	Colorectal cancer	Estimated completion, June 2013
Lappe 2012 (CAPS)[192]	RCT	Determine the effect of vitamin D_3 supplementation on all types of cancer incidence	United States	2,300	Vitamin D_3 2,000 IU qd + calcium 1,500 mg qd	Cancer	Estimated completion, June 2014
Lopez-Torres 2011[193]	RCT	Determine effectiveness of calcium and vitamin D supplementation in improving musculoskeletal function and decreasing the number of falls in older adults	Spain	704	Vitamin D 800 IU qd + calcium 1,200 mg qd	Falls, fractures, and adverse effects	Published study protocol
Manson 2012 (Vitamin D and Omega-3 Trial)[194]	RCT, 2x2 factorial design	Determine if vitamin D_3 supplementation (with or without marine omega-3 fatty acid) reduces risk for total cancer and major cardiovascular disease events	United States	20,000	Vitamin D_3 2,000 IU qd	Cancer, MI, and stroke	Published methods; estimated completion, 2017
Peto 2012 (Vitamin D and Longevity Trial [VIDAL])[195]	RCT	Determine the feasibility of a large RCT measuring the effect of oral vitamin D on morbidity and mortality in older adults	United Kingdom	20,000	Vitamin D 60,000 IU monthly	Mortality	Estimated completion, 2020
Rhodes 2009[196]	RCT	Examine effect of green tea and vitamin C on the health of human skin	United States	50	Vitamin C 100 mg with green tea qd	Skin cancer	Estimated completion, August 2012
Tran 2012[197]	RCT	Examine the effect of vitamin D supplementation on cancer incidence and overall mortality	Australia	644	Vitamin D 30,000 to 60,000 IU monthly	Cancer, mortality	Published recruitment results, 2012

Appendix C. Ongoing or Recently Completed Studies

Study	Design	Aim	Location	Number of participants	Intervention description	Relevant outcomes	2013 status
Tuomainen 2011 (Finnish Vitamin D Trial)[198]	RCT	Determine benefits and risks of vitamin D supplementation in the primary prevention of cardiovascular disease and cancer	Finland	18,000	Vitamin D_3 1,600 to 3,200 IU qd	Cardiovascular disease, MI, stroke, TIA, angina, cancer, adverse effects	Estimated completion, December 2019

Abbreviations: MI = myocardial infarction; NR = not reported; qd = once a day; RCT = randomized, controlled trial; SELECT = Selenium and Vitamin E Cancer Prevention Trial; TIA = transient ischemic attack.

Appendix D. Excluded Studies

Exclusion code
E1. Study not relevant
E2. Wrong setting
E3. Wrong population
E4. Study quality
E5. Wrong study design
E6. No relevant outcomes
E7. Precedes search period
E8. Published in a non-English language
E9. Used as a source document only
E10. Observational study reporting harms on cardiovascular disease, cancer or mortality
E11. High-dose intervention (greater than the upper tolerable limit set by the Food Nutrition Board)

1. Agler AH, Kurth T, Gaziano JM, et al. Randomised vitamin E supplementation and risk of chronic lung disease in the Women's Health Study. Thorax 2011;66(4):320-5. PMID: 21257986. **KQ3E6, KQ4E6.**
2. Albert CM, Cook NR, Gaziano JM, et al. Effect of folic acid and B vitamins on risk of cardiovascular events and total mortality among women at high risk for cardiovascular disease: a randomized trial. JAMA 2008 May 7;299(17):2027-36. PMID: 18460663. **KQ3E3.**
3. Aldosary BM, Sutter ME, Schwartz M, et al. Case series of selenium toxicity from a nutritional supplement. Clinical Toxicology: The Official Journal of the American Academy of Clinical Toxicology & European Association of Poisons Centres & Clinical Toxicologists 2012 Jan;50(1):57-64. PMID: 22165838. **KQ4E1.**
4. Algotar AM, Stratton MS, Ahmann FR, et al. Phase 3 clinical trial investigating the effect of selenium supplementation in men at high-risk for prostate cancer. Prostate 2013 Feb 15;73(3):328-35. PMID: 22887343. **KQ3E4, KQ4E4.**
5. Alkhenizan A, Hafez K. The role of vitamin E in the prevention of cancer: a meta-analysis of randomized controlled trials. Ann Saudi Med 2007 Nov;27(6):409-14. PMID: 18059122. **KQ3E9.**
6. Altaweel MM, Hanzlik RP, Ver Hoeve JN, et al. Ocular and systemic safety evaluation of calcium formate as a dietary supplement. J Ocul Pharmacol Ther 2009 Jun;25(3):223-30. PMID: 19456257. **KQ4E1.**
7. Anderson LN, Cotterchio M, Vieth R, et al. Vitamin D and calcium intakes and breast cancer risk in pre- and postmenopausal women. Am J Clin Nutr 2010 Jun;91(6):1699-707. PMID: 20392891. **KQ3E5, KQ4E1.**
8. Andreeva VA, Touvier M, Kesse-Guyot E, et al. B vitamin and/or omega-3 fatty acid supplementation and cancer: ancillary findings from the Supplementation with Folate, Vitamins B6 and B12, and/or Omega-3 fatty acids (SU.FOL.OM3) randomized trial. Arch Intern Med 2012 Apr 9;172(7):540-7. PMID: 22331983. **KQ3E5, KQ4E5.**
9. Arain MA, Abdul QA. Systematic review on "vitamin E and prevention of colorectal cancer". Pak J Pharma Sci 2010 Apr;23(2):125-30. PMID: 20363687. **KQ3E4.**
10. AREDS. A randomized, placebo-controlled, clinical trial of high-dose supplementation with vitamins C and E, beta carotene, and zinc for age-related macular degeneration and vision loss: AREDS report no. 8. Arch Ophthalmol 2001 Oct;119(10):1417-36. PMID: 11594942. **KQ2E11.**
11. AREDS. A randomized, placebo-controlled, clinical trial of high-dose supplementation with vitamins C and E and beta carotene for age-related cataract and vision loss: AREDS report no. 9. Arch Ophthalmol 2001 Oct;119(10):1439-52. PMID: 11594943. **KQ1E6, KQ2E11.**
12. Arem H, Weinstein SJ, Horst RL, et al. Serum 25-hydroxyvitamin D and risk of oropharynx and larynx cancers in finnish men. Cancer Epidemiol Biomarkers Prev 2011;20(6):1178-84. PMID: 21527582. **KQ3E1, KQ4E1.**
13. Asgari MM, Maruti SS, Kushi LH, et al. Antioxidant supplementation and risk of incident melanomas: results of a large prospective cohort study. Arch Dermatol 2009 Aug;145(8):879-82. PMID: 19687417. **KQ3E5, KQ4E5.**

Appendix D. Excluded Studies

14. Autier P, Gandini S. Vitamin D supplementation and total mortality: a meta-analysis of randomized controlled trials. Arch Intern Med 2007 Sep 10;167(16):1730-7. PMID: 17846391. **KQ3E9.**
15. Avenell A, Campbell MK, Cook JA, et al. Effect of multivitamin and multimineral supplements on morbidity from infections in older people (MAVIS trial): pragmatic, randomised, double blind, placebo controlled trial. BMJ 2005 Aug 6;331(7512):324-9. PMID: 16081445. **KQ2E6.**
16. Barengolts E. Vitamin D role and use in prediabetes. Endocr Pract 2010;16(3):476-85. PMID: 20150028. **KQ3E4, KQ4E4.**
17. Bays H, Shah A, Dong Q, et al. Extended-release niacin/laropiprant lipid-altering consistency across patient subgroups. Int J Clin Pract 2011 Apr;65(4):436-45. PMID: 21401833. **KQ3E6.**
18. Bazzano LA, Reynolds K, Holder KN, et al. Effect of folic acid supplementation on risk of cardiovascular diseases: a meta-analysis of randomized controlled trials. JAMA 2006 Dec 13;296(22):2720-6. PMID: 17164458. **KQ3E1.**
19. Beletate V, El Dib RP, Atallah AN. Zinc supplementation for the prevention of type 2 diabetes mellitus. Cochrane Database Syst Rev 2007(1):CD005525. PMID: 17253560. **KQ3E6.**
20. Bell SJ, Grochoski GT. How safe is vitamin E supplementation? Crit Rev Food Sci Nutr 2008 Sep;48(8):760-74. PMID: 18756398. **KQ4E5.**
21. Bin Q, Hu X, Cao Y, et al. The role of vitamin E (tocopherol) supplementation in the prevention of stroke. A meta-analysis of 13 randomised controlled trials. Thromb Haemost 2011 Apr;105(4):579-85. PMID: 21264448. **KQ3E9.**
22. Bjelakovic G, Nikolova D, Simonetti RG, et al. Systematic review: primary and secondary prevention of gastrointestinal cancers with antioxidant supplements. Aliment Pharmacol Ther 2008 Sep 15;28(6):689-703. PMID: 19145725. **KQ3E9.**
23. Bjelakovic G, Nikolova D, Simonetti RG, et al. Antioxidant supplements for preventing gastrointestinal cancers. Cochrane Database Syst Rev 2008(3):CD004183. PMID: 18677777. **KQ3E9.**
24. Bjelakovic G, Nikolova D, Gluud LL, et al. Antioxidant supplements for prevention of mortality in healthy participants and patients with various diseases. Cochrane Database Syst Rev 2008(2):CD007176. PMID: 18425980. **KQ3E9.**
25. Block JP. A meta-analysis raises concerns about the cardiovascular risks of calcium supplementation: Commentary. J Clin Outcomes Manage 2011;18(1):8-10. PMID: None. **KQ4E5.**
26. Blot WJ, Li JY, Taylor PR, et al. Nutrition intervention trials in Linxian, China: supplementation with specific vitamin/mineral combinations, cancer incidence, and disease-specific mortality in the general population. J Natl Cancer Inst 1993 Sep 15;85(18):1483-92. PMID: 8360931. **KQ1E2, KQ3E2.**
27. Blot WJ, Li JY, Taylor PR, et al. The Linxian trials: mortality rates by vitamin-mineral intervention group. Am J Clin Nutr 1995 Dec;62(6 Suppl):1424S-6S. PMID: 7495242. **KQ1E2, KQ3E2.**
28. Bolland MJ, Grey A, Gamble GD, et al. Risk of cardiovascular events with calcium/vitamin D: a reanalysis of the Women's Health Initiative. J Bone Miner Res 2010;25:S50. PMID: None. **KQ4E6.**
29. Bolland MJ, Avenell A, Baron JA, et al. Effect of calcium supplements on risk of myocardial infarction and cardiovascular events: meta-analysis. BMJ 2010;341:c3691. PMID: 20671013. **KQ3E9, KQ4E9.**
30. Bolland MJ, Grey A, Reid IR. Calcium supplements and cardiovascular risk. Journal of Bone & Mineral Research 2011 Apr;26(4):899-1. PMID: 21433072. **KQ3E9, KQ4E9.**
31. Bolland MJ, Grey A, Gamble GD, et al. Calcium and vitamin D supplements and health outcomes: a reanalysis of the Women's Health Initiative (WHI) limited-access data set. Am J Clin Nutr 2011 Oct;94(4):1144-9. PMID: 21880848. **KQ4E6.**
32. Bolland MJ, Grey A, Avenell A, et al. Calcium supplements with or without vitamin D and risk of cardiovascular events: reanalysis of the Women's Health Initiative limited access dataset and meta-analysis. BMJ 2011;342:d2040. PMID: 21505219. **KQ4E6.**

Appendix D. Excluded Studies

33. Brinkman MT, Karagas MR, Zens MS, et al. Minerals and vitamins and the risk of bladder cancer: results from the New Hampshire Study. Cancer Causes Control 2010 Apr;21(4):609-19. PMID: 20043202. **KQ1E1, KQ2E1, KQ4E1.**

34. Bruckert E, Labreuche J, Amarenco P. Meta-analysis of the effect of nicotinic acid alone or in combination on cardiovascular events and atherosclerosis. Atherosclerosis 2010 Jun;210(2):353-61. PMID: 20079494. **KQ3E9.**

35. Brunner RL, Wactawski-Wende J, Caan BJ, et al. The effect of calcium plus vitamin D on risk for invasive cancer: results of the Women's Health Initiative (WHI) calcium plus vitamin D randomized clinical trial. Nutrition & Cancer 2011;63(6):827-41. PMID: 21774589. **KQ4E6.**

36. Buhr G, Bales CW. Nutritional supplements for older adults: review and recommendations--Part II. J Nutr Elder 2010 Jan;29(1):42-71. PMID: 20391042. **KQ1E5, KQ3E5.**

37. Buring JE, Hennekens C. The Women's Health Study: rationale and background. J Myocardial Ischemia 1992;4(3):30-40. PMID: None. **KQ3E6, KQ4E6.**

38. Buring JE, Hennekens C. The Women's Health Study: summary of study design. J Myocardial Ischemia 1992;4(3):27-9. PMID: None. **KQ3E6, KQ4E6.**

39. Carr DR, Trevino JJ, Donnelly HB. Retinoids for chemoprophylaxis of nonmelanoma skin cancer. Dermatol Surg 2011;37(2):129-45. PMID: 21276130. **KQ3E5.**

40. Carroll C, Cooper K, Papaioannou D, et al. Supplemental calcium in the chemoprevention of colorectal cancer: a systematic review and meta-analysis. Clin Ther 2010 May;32(5):789-803. PMID: 20685491. **KQ3E9.**

41. Carroll C, Cooper K, Papaioannou D, et al. Meta-analysis: folic acid in the chemoprevention of colorectal adenomas and colorectal cancer. Aliment Pharmacol Ther 2010;31(7):708-18. PMID: 20085565. **KQ3E9.**

42. Chacko SA, Song Y, Manson JE, et al. Serum 25-hydroxyvitamin D concentrations in relation to cardiometabolic risk factors and metabolic syndrome in postmenopausal women. Am J Clin Nutr 2011;94(1):209-17. PMID: 21613558. **KQ3E1, KQ4E1.**

43. Chae CU, Albert CM, Moorthy MV, et al. Vitamin E supplementation and the risk of heart failure in women. Circ Heart Fail 2012 Mar 1;5(2):176-82. PMID: 22438520. **KQ4E6.**

44. Chan AL, Leung HW, Wang SF. Multivitamin supplement use and risk of breast cancer: a meta-analysis. Ann Pharmacother 2011 Apr;45(4):476-84. PMID: 21487086. **KQ2E1, KQ3E1.**

45. Chen P, Hu P, Xie D, et al. Meta-analysis of vitamin D, calcium and the prevention of breast cancer. Breast Cancer Res Treat 2010 Jun;121(2):469-77. PMID: 19851861. **KQ3E1.**

46. Chlebowski RT, Pettinger M, Kooperberg C. Caution in reinterpreting the Women's Health Initiative (WHI) calcium and vitamin D trial breast cancer results. Am J Clin Nutr 2012;95(1):258-9. PMID: 22189262. **KQ3E6, KQ4E6.**

47. Christen WG, Glynn RJ, Sesso HD, et al. Vitamins E and C and medical record-confirmed age-related macular degeneration in a randomized trial of male physicians. Ophthalmology 2012 Aug;119(8):1642-9. PMID: 22503302. **KQ3E6, KQ4E6.**

48. Chung, M, Balk, EM, Brendel, M, et al. Vitamin D and calcium: a systematic review of health outcomes. AHRQ Publication No. 09-E015. Rockville, MD: Agency for Healthcare Research and Quality; 2009. PMID: 20629479. **KQ3E9, KQ4E9.**

49. Clark L, Krongrad A, Dalkin B, et al. Decreased incidence of prostate cancer with selenium supplementation: 1983-96 results of a double-blind cancer prevention trial. Eur J Cancer Prev 1997;6(5):497-8. PMID: None. **KQ3E9.**

50. Clarke R, Lewington S, Sherliker P, et al. Effects of B-vitamins on plasma homocysteine concentrations and on risk of cardiovascular disease and dementia. Curr Opin Clin Nutr Metab Care 2007 Jan;10(1):32-9. PMID: 17143052. **KQ3E3, KQ4E3.**

51. Clarke R, Halsey J, Lewington S, et al. Effects of lowering homocysteine levels with B vitamins on cardiovascular disease, cancer, and cause-specific mortality: Meta-analysis of 8 randomized trials involving 37 485 individuals. Arch Intern Med 2010 Oct 11;170(18):1622-31. PMID: 20937919. **KQ3E3.**

Appendix D. Excluded Studies

52. Clarke R, Halsey J, Bennett D, et al. Homocysteine and vascular disease: review of published results of the homocysteine-lowering trials. J Inherit Metab Dis 2011 Feb;34(1):83-91. PMID: 21069462. **KQ3E3.**

53. Cole BF, Baron JA, Sandler RS, et al. Folic acid for the prevention of colorectal adenomas: a randomized clinical trial. JAMA 2007 Jun 6;297(21):2351-9. PMID: 17551129. **KQ4E6.**

54. Cook LS, Neilson HK, Lorenzetti DL, et al. A systematic literature review of vitamin D and ovarian cancer. Am J Obstet Gynecol 2010 Jul;203(1):70-8. PMID: 20227054. **KQ3E1.**

55. Cook NR, Le IM, Manson JE, et al. Effects of beta-carotene supplementation on cancer incidence by baseline characteristics in the Physicians' Health Study (United States). Cancer Causes Control 2000 Aug;11(7):617-26. PMID: 10977106. **KQ4E6.**

56. Cooper K, Squires H, Carroll C, et al. Chemoprevention of colorectal cancer: systematic review and economic evaluation. Health Technol Assess 2010 Jun;14(32):1-206. PMID: 20594533. **KQ1E9, KQ3E9.**

57. Coulter ID, Hardy ML, Morton SC, et al. Antioxidants vitamin C and vitamin e for the prevention and treatment of cancer. J Gen Intern Med 2006 Jul;21(7):735-44. PMID: 16808775. **KQ3E9.**

58. Cranney, A, Horsley, T, O'Donnell, S, et al. Effectiveness and safety of vitamin D in relation to bone health. AHRQ Publication No. 07-E013. Rockville, MD: Agency for Healthcare Research and Quality; 2007. PMID: 18088161. **KQ4E9.**

59. Davey SG, Ebrahim S. Folate supplementation and cardiovascular disease. Lancet 2005 Nov 12;366(9498):1679-81. PMID: 16291049. **KQ3E5, KQ4E5.**

60. de Gaetano G. Low-dose aspirin and vitamin E in people at cardiovascular risk: a randomised trial in general practice. Collaborative Group of the Primary Prevention Project. Lancet 2001 Jan 13;357(9250):89-95. PMID: 11197445. **KQ3E3.**

61. Dennert G, Zwahlen M, Brinkman M, et al. Selenium for preventing cancer. Cochrane Database Syst Rev 2011;5:CD005195. PMID: 21563143. **KQ3E9.**

62. Dietrich M, Jacques PF, Pencina MJ, et al. Vitamin E supplement use and the incidence of cardiovascular disease and all-cause mortality in the Framingham Heart Study: Does the underlying health status play a role? Atherosclerosis 2009 Aug;205(2):549-53. PMID: 19195657. **KQ3E5, KQ4E5.**

63. Dotan Y, Pinchuk I, Lichtenberg D, et al. Decision analysis supports the paradigm that indiscriminate supplementation of vitamin E does more harm than good. Arterioscler Thromb Vasc Biol 2009 Sep;29(9):1304-9. PMID: 19286632. **KQ4E5.**

64. Driscoll MS, Kwon EK, Skupsky H, et al. Nutrition and the deleterious side effects of nutritional supplements. Clin Dermatol 2010 Jul;28(4):371-9. PMID: 20620752. **KQ4E5.**

65. Druesne-Pecollo N, Latino-Martel P, Norat T, et al. Beta-carotene supplementation and cancer risk: a systematic review and metaanalysis of randomized controlled trials. Int J Cancer 2010 Jul 1;127(1):172-84. PMID: 19876916. **KQ3E9.**

66. Duffield-Lillico AJ, Reid ME, Turnbull BW, et al. Baseline characteristics and the effect of selenium supplementation on cancer incidence in a randomized clinical trial: a summary report of the Nutritional Prevention of Cancer Trial. Cancer Epidemiol Biomarkers Prev 2002 Jul;11(7):630-9. PMID: 12101110. **KQ4E6.**

67. Duffield-Lillico AJ, Slate EH, Reid ME, et al. Selenium supplementation and secondary prevention of nonmelanoma skin cancer in a randomized trial. J Natl Cancer Inst 2003 Oct 1;95(19):1477-81. PMID: 14519754. **KQ3E3.**

68. Duffield-Lillico AJ, Dalkin BL, Reid ME, et al. Selenium supplementation, baseline plasma selenium status and incidence of prostate cancer: an analysis of the complete treatment period of the Nutritional Prevention of Cancer Trial. BJU Int 2003 May;91(7):608-12. PMID: 12699469. **KQ4E6.**

69. Durga J, Bots ML, Schouten EG, et al. Effect of 3 y of folic acid supplementation on the progression of carotid intima-media thickness and carotid arterial stiffness in older adults. Am J Clin Nutr 2011 May;93(5):941-9. PMID: 21430116. **KQ3E1, KQ4E1.**

Appendix D. Excluded Studies

70. Earnest CP, Kupper JS, Thompson AM, et al. Complementary effects of multivitamin and omega-3 fatty acid supplementation on indices of cardiovascular health in individuals with elevated homocysteine. Int J Vitam Nutr Res 2012 Feb;82(1):41-52. PMID: 22811376. **KQ1E6, KQ2E6.**
71. Ebbing M, Bonaa KH, Nygard O, et al. Cancer incidence and mortality after treatment with folic acid and vitamin B12. JAMA 2009 Nov 18;302(19):2119-26. PMID: 19920236. **KQ3E3, KQ4E3.**
72. Ebbing M, Bonaa KH, Arnesen E, et al. Combined analyses and extended follow-up of two randomized controlled homocysteine-lowering B-vitamin trials. J Intern Med 2010 Oct;268(4):367-82. PMID: 20698927. **KQ3E3, KQ4E3.**
73. Edvardsen K, Veierod MB, Brustad M, et al. Vitamin D-effective solar UV radiation, dietary vitamin D and breast cancer risk. Int J Cancer 2011 Mar 15;128(6):1425-33. PMID: 20473950. **KQ3E1, KQ4E1.**
74. Ezzedine K, Latreille J, Kesse-Guyot E, et al. Incidence of skin cancers during 5-year follow-up after stopping antioxidant vitamins and mineral supplementation. Eur J Cancer 2010 Dec;46(18):3316-22. PMID: 20605091. **KQ2E6.**
75. Fenton A, Panay N. Calcium supplementation: is there a cardiovascular risk? Climacteric 2011 Feb;14(1):1-2. PMID: 21235419. **KQ4E5.**
76. Fife J, Raniga S, Hider PN, et al. Folic acid supplementation and colorectal cancer risk: a meta-analysis. Colorectal Dis 2011 Feb;13(2):132-7. PMID: 19863600. **KQ3E4.**
77. Figueiredo JC, Mott LA, Giovannucci E, et al. Folic acid and prevention of colorectal adenomas: a combined analysis of randomized clinical trials. Int J Cancer 2011 Jul 1;129(1):192-203. PMID: 21170989. **KQ3E6.**
78. Ford JA, MacLennan G, Bolland MJ, et al. Vitamin d supplementation prevents cardiac failure; MRC record trial analysis, systematic review and meta-analysis. Circulation 2012;126:A18397. PMID: None. **KQ4E6.**
79. Forman MR, Levin B. Calcium plus vitamin D3 supplementation and colorectal cancer in women. New Engl J Med 2006;354(7):752-4. PMID: 19276452. **KQ3E5, KQ4E5.**
80. Frieling UM, Schaumberg DA, Kupper TS, et al. A randomized, 12-year primary-prevention trial of beta carotene supplementation for nonmelanoma skin cancer in the physician's health study. Arch Dermatol 2000 Feb;136(2):179-84. PMID: 10677093. **KQ3E6, KQ4E6.**
81. Fritz H, Kennedy D, Fernandes R, et al. Selenium and lung cancer: A systematic review. J Soc Integr Oncol 2010;8(4):203-4. PMID: None. **KQ3E4.**
82. Fritz H, Kennedy D, Fernandes R, et al. Vitamin D and lung cancer: A systematic review. J Soc Integr Oncol 2010;8(4):205. PMID: None. **KQ3E4.**
83. Fu T, Tang JY, Leblanc E, et al. Calcium plus vitamin D supplementation and the risk of nonmelanoma and melanoma skin cancer. J Invest Dermatol 2011;131(Suppl 1):S35. PMID: None. **KQ4E6.**
84. Garland CF, French CB, Baggerly LL, et al. Vitamin D supplement doses and serum 25-hydroxyvitamin D in the range associated with cancer prevention. Anticancer Res 2011 Feb;31(2):607-11. PMID: 21378345. **KQ3E1, KQ4E1.**
85. Geleijnse JM. Vitamin D and the prevention of hypertension and cardiovascular diseases: a review of the current evidence. Am J Hypertens 2011 Mar;24(3):253-62. PMID: 20847727. **KQ3E5, KQ4E5.**
86. Gepner AD, Ramamurthy R, Krueger DC, et al. A prospective randomized controlled trial of the effects of vitamin D supplementation on cardiovascular disease risk. PLoS ONE 2012;7(5):e36617. PMID: 22586483. **KQ3E6, KQ4E6.**
87. Gerss J, Kopcke W. The questionable association of vitamin E supplementation and mortality--inconsistent results of different meta-analytic approaches. Cell Mol Biol 2009;55:Suppl-20. PMID: 19267994. **KQ4E1.**
88. Goodman GE, Thornquist MD, Balmes J, et al. The Beta-Carotene and Retinol Efficacy Trial: incidence of lung cancer and cardiovascular disease mortality during 6-year follow-up after stopping beta-carotene and retinol supplements. J Natl Cancer Inst 2004 Dec 1;96(23):1743-50. PMID: 15572756. **KQ4E6.**
89. Goodman PJ, Hartline JA, Tangen CM, et al. Moving a randomized clinical trial into an observational cohort. Clin Trials 2013;10(1):131-42. PMID: 23064404. **KQ3E6, KQ4E6.**

Appendix D. Excluded Studies

90. Greenberg ER, Baron JA, Tosteson TD, et al. A clinical trial of antioxidant vitamins to prevent colorectal adenoma. Polyp Prevention Study Group. N Engl J Med 1994 Jul 21;331(3):141-7. PMID: 8008027. **KQ1E6, KQ3E6.**

91. Greenberg ER, Baron JA, Karagas MR, et al. Mortality associated with low plasma concentration of beta carotene and the effect of oral supplementation. JAMA 1996 Mar 6;275(9):699-703. PMID: 8594267. **KQ4E6.**

92. Hankey GJ, Eikelboom J, Yi Q, et al. B vitamin supplementation and incidence of cancer in patients with previous stroke or transient ischemic attack (TIA): Results of a randomised trial. Int J Stroke 2012;7(Suppl 1):43. PMID: None. **KQ1E3, KQ2E3.**

93. Hankey GJ, Eikelboom JW, Yi Q, et al. Treatment with B vitamins and incidence of cancer in patients with previous stroke or transient ischemic attack: results of a randomized placebo-controlled trial. Stroke 2012 Jun;43(6):1572-7. PMID: 22474057. **KQ1E3, KQ2E6.**

94. Hatfield DL, Gladyshev VN. The Outcome of Selenium and Vitamin E Cancer Prevention Trial (SELECT) reveals the need for better understanding of selenium biology. Mol Interv 2009 Feb;9(1):18-21. PMID: 19299660. **KQ3E5.**

95. Hatzitolios A, Iliadis F, Katsiki N, et al. Is the anti-hypertensive effect of dietary supplements via aldehydes reduction evidence based? A systematic review. Clin Exp Hypertens 2008 Oct;30(7):628-39. PMID: 18855266. **KQ1E4.**

96. Hayden KM, Welsh-Bohmer KA, Wengreen HJ, et al. Risk of mortality with vitamin E supplements: the Cache County study. Am J Med 2007 Feb;120(2):180-4. PMID: 17275460. **KQ3E5, KQ4E5.**

97. Hemila H, Kaprio J. Vitamin E supplementation may transiently increase tuberculosis risk in males who smoke heavily and have high dietary vitamin C intake. Br J Nutr 2008 Oct;100(4):896-902. PMID: 18279551. **KQ3E6, KQ4E6.**

98. Hemilä H, Kaprio J. Vitamin E supplementation may transiently increase tuberculosis risk in males who smoke heavily and have high dietary vitamin C intake. Br J Nutr 2008;100(4):896-902. PMID: 18279551. **KQ3E6, KQ4E6.**

99. Hercberg S, Czernichow S, Galan P. Antioxidant vitamins and minerals in prevention of cancers: lessons from the SU.VI.MAX study. Br J Nutr 2006 Aug;96:Suppl-30. PMID: 16923246. **KQ2E6.**

100. Hercberg S, Ezzedine K, Guinot C, et al. Antioxidant supplementation increases the risk of skin cancers in women but not in men. J Nutr 2007 Sep;137(9):2098-105. PMID: 17709449. **KQ2E6.**

101. Hercberg S, Kesse-Guyot E, Druesne-Pecollo N, et al. Incidence of cancers, ischemic cardiovascular diseases and mortality during 5-year follow-up after stopping antioxidant vitamins and minerals supplements: a postintervention follow-up in the SU.VI.MAX Study. Int J Cancer 2010 Oct 15;127(8):1875-81. PMID: 20104528. **KQ2E6.**

102. Hernaandez J, Syed S, Weiss G, et al. The modulation of prostate cancer risk with alpha-tocopherol: a pilot randomized, controlled clinical trial. J Urol 2005 Aug;174(2):519-22. PMID: 16006884. **KQ3E6.**

103. Hernandez J, Syed S, Weiss G, et al. The modulation of prostate cancer risk with a-tocopherol: a pilot randomized, controlled clinical trial. J Urol 2005;174(2):519-22. PMID: 16006884. **KQ3E6, KQ4E6.**

104. Hsia J, Heiss G, Ren H, et al. Calcium/vitamin D supplementation and cardiovascular events. Circulation 2007 Feb 20;115(7):846-54. PMID: 17309935. **KQ4E6.**

105. Ishitani K, Lin J, Manson JE, et al. A prospective study of multivitamin supplement use and risk of breast cancer. Am J Epidemiol 2008;167(10):1197-206. PMID: 18344515. **KQ1E5, KQ2E6.**

106. Jackson RD, LaCroix AZ, Cauley JA, et al. The Women's Health Initiative calcium-vitamin D trial: overview and baseline characteristics of participants. Ann Epidemiol 2003 Oct;13(9 Suppl):S98-106. PMID: 14575942. **KQ3E6.**

107. Jiang L, Yang KH, Tian JH, et al. Efficacy of antioxidant vitamins and selenium supplement in prostate cancer prevention: a meta-analysis of randomized controlled trials. Nutr Cancer 2010 Aug;62(6):719-27. PMID: 20661819. **KQ3E9.**

Appendix D. Excluded Studies

108. Johnson AR, Munoz A, Gottlieb JL, et al. High dose zinc increases hospital admissions due to genitourinary complications. J Urol 2007 Feb;177(2):639-43. PMID: 17222649. **KQ4E11.**

109. Kataja-Tuomola MK, Kontto JP, Mannisto S, et al. Intake of antioxidants and risk of type 2 diabetes in a cohort of male smokers. Eur J Clin Nutr 2011;65(5):590-7. PMID: 21245884. **KQ3E5.**

110. Kennedy DA, Stern SJ, Moretti M, et al. Folate intake and the risk of colorectal cancer: a systematic review and meta-analysis. Cancer Epidemiol 2011 Feb;35(1):2-10. PMID: 21177150. **KQ3E4.**

111. Kesse-Guyot E, Touvier M, Henegar A, et al. Higher adherence to French dietary guidelines and chronic diseases in the prospective SU.VI.MAX cohort. Eur J Clin Nutr 2011 Aug;65(8):887-94. PMID: 21559045. **KQ3E1, KQ4E1.**

112. Kirsh VA, Hayes RB, Mayne ST, et al. Supplemental and dietary vitamin E, beta-carotene, and vitamin C intakes and prostate cancer risk. J Natl Cancer Inst 2006 Feb 15;98(4):245-54. PMID: 16478743. **KQ3E5, KQ4E5.**

113. Kristal AR, Arnold KB, Neuhouser ML, et al. Diet, supplement use, and prostate cancer risk: results from the prostate cancer prevention trial. Am J Epidemiol 2010 Sep 1;172(5):566-77. PMID: 20693267. **KQ3E5.**

114. Larsson SC, Wolk A. Magnesium intake and risk of type 2 diabetes: a meta-analysis. J Intern Med 2007 Aug;262(2):208-14. PMID: 17645588. **KQ3E1, KQ4E1.**

115. Larsson SC, Akesson A, Bergkvist L, et al. Multivitamin use and breast cancer incidence in a prospective cohort of Swedish women. Am J Clin Nutr 2010 May;91(5):1268-72. PMID: 20335555. **KQ2E10.**

116. Larsson SC, Orsini N, Wolk A. Vitamin B6 and risk of colorectal cancer: a meta-analysis of prospective studies. JAMA 2010 Mar 17;303(11):1077-83. PMID: 20233826. **KQ3E1.**

117. Lawson KA, Wright ME, Subar A, et al. Multivitamin use and risk of prostate cancer in the National Institutes of Health-AARP Diet and Health Study. J Natl Cancer Inst 2007 May 16;99(10):754-64. PMID: 17505071. **KQ2E5, KQ3E5, KQ4E5.**

118. Ledesma MC, Jung-Hynes B, Schmit TL, et al. Selenium and vitamin E for prostate cancer: Post SELECT (selenium and vitamin E cancer prevention trial) status. Mol Med 2011;17(1-2):134-43. PMID: 20882260. **KQ3E5.**

119. Lee JE, Li H, Chan AT, et al. Circulating levels of vitamin D and colon and rectal cancer: the Physicians' Health Study and a meta-analysis of prospective studies. Cancer Prev Res 2011 May;4(5):735-43. PMID: 21430073. **KQ3E1.**

120. Lee JE, Willett WC, Fuchs CS, et al. Folate intake and risk of colorectal cancer and adenoma: modification by time. Am J Clin Nutr 2011 Apr;93(4):817-25. PMID: 21270374. **KQ3E5, KQ4E6.**

121. Lee M, Hong KS, Chang SC, et al. Efficacy of homocysteine-lowering therapy with folic Acid in stroke prevention: a meta-analysis. Stroke 2010 Jun;41(6):1205-12. PMID: 20413740. **KQ3E3.**

122. Leppala JM, Virtamo J, Fogelholm R, et al. Controlled trial of alpha-tocopherol and beta-carotene supplements on stroke incidence and mortality in male smokers. Arterioscler Thromb Vasc Biol 2000 Jan;20(1):230-5. PMID: 10634823. **KQ3E6.**

123. Lewis JR, Calver J, Zhu K, et al. Calcium supplementation and the risks of atherosclerotic vascular disease in older women: results of a 5-year RCT and a 4.5-year follow-up. J Bone Miner Res 2011 Jan;26(1):35-41. PMID: 20614474. **KQ3E3, KQ4E3.**

124. Li J, Hou Z. Whether vitamin E supplements can decrease the risk of prostate cancer: Meta analysis. J Clin Rehab Tissue Eng Res 2010;14(28):5177-80. PMID: None. **KQ3E8.**

125. Li K, Kaaks R, Linseisen J, et al. Associations of dietary calcium intake and calcium supplementation with myocardial infarction and stroke risk and overall cardiovascular mortality in the Heidelberg cohort of the European Prospective Investigation into Cancer and Nutrition study (EPIC-Heidelberg). Heart 2012 Jun;98(12):920-5. PMID: 22626900. **KQ3E5, KQ4E5.**

126. Li K, Kaaks R, Linseisen J, et al. Vitamin/mineral supplementation and cancer, cardiovascular, and all-cause mortality in a German prospective cohort (EPIC-Heidelberg). Eur J Nutr 2012 Jun;51(4):407-13. **KQ1E5, KQ2E6.**

Appendix D. Excluded Studies

127. Lin J, Cook NR, Albert C, et al. Vitamins C and E and beta carotene supplementation and cancer risk: a randomized controlled trial. J Natl Cancer Inst 2009 Jan 7;101(1):14-23. PMID: 19116389. **KQ3E3.**
128. Loke YK, Price D, Derry S, et al. Case reports of suspected adverse drug reactions--systematic literature survey of follow-up. BMJ 2006 Feb 11;332(7537):335-9. PMID: 16421149. **KQ2E1, KQ4E1.**
129. Lonn E, Bosch J, Yusuf S, et al. Effects of long-term vitamin E supplementation on cardiovascular events and cancer: a randomized controlled trial. JAMA 2005 Mar 16;293(11):1338-47. PMID: 15769967. **KQ3E3.**
130. Lopez-Torres HJ, ANVITAD Group. Prevention of falls and fractures in old people by administration of calcium and vitamin D. randomized clinical trial. BMC Public Health 2011;11:910. PMID: 22151975. **KQ4E9.**
131. Lotan Y, Goodman P, Youssef R, et al. Evaluation of vitamin E and selenium supplementation on the prevention of bladder cancer in swog-coordinated select. J Urol 2012;187(6):2005-10. PMID: 22498220. **KQ4E6.**
132. Magliano D, McNeil J, Branley P, et al. The Melbourne Atherosclerosis Vitamin E Trial (MAVET): a study of high dose vitamin E in smokers. Eur J Cardiovasc Prev Rehabil 2006 Jun;13(3):341-7. PMID: 16926662. **KQ3E6.**
133. Malila N, Virtamo J, Virtanen M, et al. The effect of alpha-tocopherol and beta-carotene supplementation on colorectal adenomas in middle-aged male smokers. Cancer Epidemiol Biomarkers Prev 1999 Jun;8(6):489-93. PMID: 10385137. **KQ3E6, KQ4E6.**
134. Manson JE, Bassuk SS, Lee IM, et al. The VITamin D and OmegA-3 TriaL (VITAL): rationale and design of a large randomized controlled trial of vitamin D and marine omega-3 fatty acid supplements for the primary prevention of cancer and cardiovascular disease. Contemp Clin Trials 2012 Jan;33(1):159-71. PMID: 21986389. **KQ3E9, KQ4E9.**
135. Margolis KL, Ray RM, Van HL, et al. Effect of calcium and vitamin D supplementation on blood pressure: the Women's Health Initiative Randomized Trial. Hypertension 2008 Nov;52(5):847-55. PMID: 18824662. **KQ3E6.**
136. Margolis KL, Ray RM, Kerby TJ. The womens health initiative calcium/vitamin D trial. Hypertension 2011;57(4):e14. PMID: 21357276. **KQ3E5.**
137. Mark SD, Wang W, Fraumeni JF, Jr., et al. Do nutritional supplements lower the risk of stroke or hypertension? Epidemiology 1998 Jan;9(1):9-15. PMID: 9430262. **KQ1E2, KQ3E2.**
138. Martini LA, Catania AS, Ferreira SRG. Role of vitamins and minerals in prevention and management of type 2 diabetes mellitus. Nutr Rev 2010;68(6):341-54. PMID: 20536779. **KQ3E5.**
139. Mazdak H, Zia H. Vitamin E reduces superficial bladder cancer recurrence: A randomized controlled trial. Int J Prev Med 2012;3(2):110-5. PMID: 22347607. **KQ3E6, KQ4E6.**
140. McCullough ML, Bandera EV, Moore DF, et al. Vitamin D and calcium intake in relation to risk of endometrial cancer: a systematic review of the literature. Prev Med 2008 Apr;46(4):298-302. PMID: 18155758. **KQ3E9.**
141. McNeil JJ, Robman L, Tikellis G, et al. Vitamin E supplementation and cataract: randomized controlled trial. Ophthalmology 2004 Jan;111(1):75-84. PMID: 14711717. **KQ3E6, KQ4E6.**
142. Meydani SN, Meydani M, Blumberg JB, et al. Assessment of the safety of supplementation with different amounts of vitamin E in healthy older adults. Am J Clin Nutr 1998 Aug;68(2):311-8. PMID: 9701188. **KQ3E6, KQ4E6.**
143. Michaud DS. Vitamin D and pancreatic cancer risk in the alpha-tocopherol, beta-carotene cancer prevention cohort. Cancer Res 2006 Oct 15;66(20):9802-3. PMID: 17047039. **KQ3E5, KQ4E5.**
144. Miller ER, III, Pastor-Barriuso R, Dalal D, et al. Meta-analysis: high-dosage vitamin E supplementation may increase all-cause mortality. Ann Intern Med 2005 Jan 4;142(1):37-46. PMID: 15537682. **KQ4E9.**
145. Miller ER, III, Juraschek S, Pastor-Barriuso R, et al. Meta-analysis of folic acid supplementation trials on risk of cardiovascular disease and risk interaction with baseline homocysteine levels. Am J Cardiol 2010 Aug 15;106(4):517-27. PMID: 20691310. **KQ3E9.**

Appendix D. Excluded Studies

146. Moon TE, Levine N, Cartmel B, et al. Effect of retinol in preventing squamous cell skin cancer in moderate-risk subjects: a randomized, double-blind, controlled trial. Southwest Skin Cancer Prevention Study Group. Cancer Epidemiol Biomarkers Prev 1997 Nov;6(11):949-56. PMID: 9367069. **KQ3E6.**

147. Mursu J, Robien K, Harnack LJ, et al. Dietary supplements and mortality rate in older women: The Iowa Women's Health Study. Arch Intern Med 2011;171(18):1625-33. PMID: 21987192. **KQ1E6, KQ2E6, KQ3E6, KQ4E6.**

148. Myung SK, Kim Y, Ju W, et al. Effects of antioxidant supplements on cancer prevention: Meta-analysis of randomized controlled trials. Ann Oncol 2010;21(1):166-79. PMID: 19622597. **KQ3E9.**

149. Ntaios G, Savopoulos C, Grekas D, et al. The controversial role of B-vitamins in cardiovascular risk: An update. Arch Cardiovasc Dis 2009;102(12):847-54. PMID: 19963194. **KQ3E5, KQ4E5.**

150. Omenn GS, Goodman GE, Thornquist M, et al. Long-term vitamin A does not produce clinically significant hypertriglyceridemia: results from CARET, the beta-carotene and retinol efficacy trial. Cancer Epidemiol Biomarkers Prev 1994 Dec;3(8):711-3. PMID: 7881345. **KQ3E6, KQ4E6.**

151. Omenn GS, Goodman GE, Thornquist MD, et al. Risk factors for lung cancer and for intervention effects in CARET, the Beta-Carotene and Retinol Efficacy Trial. J Natl Cancer Inst 1996 Nov 6;88(21):1550-9. PMID: 8901853. **KQ4E6.**

152. Peters U, Littman AJ, Kristal AR, et al. Vitamin E and selenium supplementation and risk of prostate cancer in the Vitamins and lifestyle (VITAL) study cohort. Cancer Causes Control 2008 Feb;19(1):75-87. PMID: 17943452. **KQ3E5.**

153. Pilz S, Tomaschitz A, Drechsler C, et al. Vitamin D supplementation: a promising approach for the prevention and treatment of strokes. Curr Drug Targets 2011 Jan;12(1):88-96. PMID: 20795935. **KQ3E5.**

154. Pittas AG, Lau J, Hu FB, et al. The role of vitamin D and calcium in type 2 diabetes. A systematic review and meta-analysis. J Clin Endocrinol Metab 2007 Jun;92(6):2017-29. PMID: 17389701. **KQ3E9.**

155. Pittas AG, Chung M, Trikalinos T, et al. Systematic review: Vitamin D and cardiometabolic outcomes. Ann Intern Med 2010 Mar 2;152(5):307-14. PMID: 20194237. **KQ3E9.**

156. Prince RL, Devine A, Dhaliwal SS, et al. Effects of calcium supplementation on clinical fracture and bone structure: results of a 5-year, double-blind, placebo-controlled trial in elderly women. Arch Intern Med 2006 Apr 24;166(8):869-75. PMID: 16636212. **KQ4E6.**

157. Rapola JM, Virtamo J, Haukka JK, et al. Effect of vitamin E and beta carotene on the incidence of angina pectoris. A randomized, double-blind, controlled trial. JAMA 1996 Mar 6;275(9):693-8. PMID: 8594266. **KQ3E6.**

158. Rapola JM, Virtamo J, Ripatti S, et al. Randomised trial of alpha-tocopherol and beta-carotene supplements on incidence of major coronary events in men with previous myocardial infarction. Lancet 1997 Jun 14;349(9067):1715-20. PMID: 9193380. **KQ3E3, KQ4E3.**

159. Rayman MP, Blundell-Pound G, Pastor-Barriuso R, et al. A randomized trial of selenium supplementation and risk of type-2 diabetes, as assessed by plasma adiponectin. PLoS ONE 2012;7(9):e45269. PMID: 16636212. **KQ3E6.**

160. Reid IR, Mason B, Horne A, et al. Effects of calcium supplementation on serum lipid concentrations in normal older women: a randomized controlled trial. Am J Med 2002 Apr 1;112(5):343-7. PMID: 11904107. **KQ3E6.**

161. Reid IR, Bolland MJ. Calcium supplementation and vascular disease. Climacteric 2008 Aug;11(4):280-6. PMID: 18645693. **KQ4E5.**

162. Reid IR, Ames R, Mason B, et al. Randomized controlled trial of calcium supplementation in healthy, nonosteoporotic, older men. Arch Intern Med 2008 Nov 10;168(20):2276-82. PMID: 19001206. **KQ4E6.**

163. Reid IR, Bolland MJ, Avenell A, et al. Cardiovascular effects of calcium supplementation. Osteoporos Int 2011 Jun;22(6):1649-58. PMID: 21409434. **KQ3E5, KQ4E5.**

Appendix D. Excluded Studies

164. Reid ME, Duffield-Lillico AJ, Sunga A, et al. Selenium supplementation and colorectal adenomas: an analysis of the nutritional prevention of cancer trial. Int J Cancer 2006 Apr 1;118(7):1777-81. PMID: 16217756. **KQ3E6.**
165. Reid ME, Duffield-Lillico AJ, Slate E, et al. The nutritional prevention of cancer: 400 mcg per day selenium treatment. Nutr Cancer 2008;60(2):155-63. PMID: 18444146. **KQ4E6.**
166. Rexrode KM, Lee IM, Cook NR, et al. Baseline characteristics of participants in the Women's Health Study. J Womens Health Gend Based Med 2000 Jan;9(1):19-27. PMID: 10718501. **KQ3E6, KQ4E6.**
167. Rogovik AL, Vohra S, Goldman RD. Safety considerations and potential interactions of vitamins: should vitamins be considered drugs? Ann Pharmacother 2010 Feb;44(2):311-24. PMID: 20040703. **KQ4E11.**
168. Rohan TE, Negassa A, Chlebowski RT, et al. A randomized controlled trial of calcium plus vitamin D supplementation and risk of benign proliferative breast disease. Breast Cancer Res Treat 2009 Jul;116(2):339-50. PMID: 18853250. **KQ3E6.**
169. Sacco M, Pellegrini F, Roncaglioni MC, et al. Primary prevention of cardiovascular events with low-dose aspirin and vitamin E in type 2 diabetic patients: results of the Primary Prevention Project (PPP) trial. Diabetes Care 2003 Dec;26(12):3264-72. PMID: 14633812. **KQ3E3.**
170. Salehpour A, Shidfar F, Hosseinpanah F, et al. Vitamin D3 and the risk of CVD in overweight and obese women: A randomised controlled trial. Br J Nutr 2012;108(10):1866-73. PMID: 22317756. **KQ3E6, KQ4E6.**
171. Satia JA, Littman A, Slatore CG, et al. Long-term use of beta-carotene, retinol, lycopene, and lutein supplements and lung cancer risk: results from the VITamins And Lifestyle (VITAL) study. Am J Epidemiol 2009 Apr 1;169(7):815-28. PMID: 19208726. **KQ4E10.**
172. Sauer J, Mason JB, Choi SW. Too much folate: A risk factor for cancer and cardiovascular disease? Curr Opin Clin Nutr Metab Care 2009;12(1):30-6. PMID: 19057184. **KQ4E5.**
173. Schulze MB, Schulz M, Heidemann C, et al. Fiber and magnesium intake and incidence of type 2 diabetes: a prospective study and meta-analysis. Arch Intern Med 2007 May 14;167(9):956-65. PMID: 17502538. **KQ3E1, KQ4E1.**
174. Shah SM, Carey IM, Harris T, et al. Calcium supplementation, cardiovascular disease and mortality in older women. Pharmacoepidemiol Drug Saf 2010 Jan;19(1):59-64. PMID: 19757413. **KQ3E5, KQ4E5.**
175. Slatore CG, Littman AJ, Au DH, et al. Long-term use of supplemental multivitamins, vitamin C, vitamin E, and folate does not reduce the risk of lung cancer. Am J Respir Crit Care Med 2008 Mar 1;177(5):524-30. PMID: 17989343. **KQ1E5, KQ3E5.**
176. Song Y, Cook NR, Christine MA, et al. Effects of vitamins C and E and beta-carotene on the incidence of type 2 diabetes mellitus in the Women's Antioxidant Cardiovascular Study randomized controlled trial. Am J Epidemiol 2008;167(Suppl 11):S146. PMID: None. **KQ3E3.**
177. Sood A, Arora R. Mechanisms of flushing due to niacin and abolition of these effects. J Clin Hypertens 2009 Nov;11(11):685-9. PMID: 19878384. **KQ4E5.**
178. Stampfer M, Rimm E, Willett W. Folate supplementation and cardiovascular disease. Lancet 2006;367(9518):1237-8. PMID: 16631874. **KQ3E5, KQ4E5.**
179. Stranges S, Marshall JR, Trevisan M, et al. Effects of selenium supplementation on cardiovascular disease incidence and mortality: secondary analyses in a randomized clinical trial. Am J Epidemiol 2006 Apr 15;163(8):694-9. PMID: 16495471. **KQ4E6.**
180. Stratton J, Godwin M. The effect of supplemental vitamins and minerals on the development of prostate cancer: a systematic review and meta-analysis. Fam Pract 2011 Jun;28(3):243-52. PMID: 21273283. **KQ1E9.**
181. Stratton MS, Reid ME, Schwartzberg G, et al. Selenium and prevention of prostate cancer in high-risk men: the Negative Biopsy Study. Anticancer Drugs 2003 Sep;14(8):589-94. PMID: 14501380. **KQ3E4, KQ4E4.**

Appendix D. Excluded Studies

182. Tanvetyanon T, Bepler G. Beta-carotene in multivitamins and the possible risk of lung cancer among smokers versus former smokers: a meta-analysis and evaluation of national brands. Cancer 2008 Jul 1;113(1):150-7. PMID: 18429004. **KQ3E9, KQ4E9.**
183. Taylor PR, Li B, Dawsey SM, et al. Prevention of esophageal cancer: the nutrition intervention trials in Linxian, China. Linxian Nutrition Intervention Trials Study Group. Cancer Res 1994 Apr 1;54(7 Suppl):2029s-31s. PMID: 8137333. **KQ1E2, KQ3E2.**
184. Thomas J. Multivitamins associated with increased cancer outcomes and all-cause mortality. Aust J Pharm 2010;91(1081):74. PMID: None. **KQ2E5, KQ3E5, KQ4E5.**
185. Tornwall ME, Virtamo J, Korhonen PA, et al. Postintervention effect of alpha tocopherol and beta carotene on different strokes: a 6-year follow-up of the Alpha Tocopherol, Beta Carotene Cancer Prevention Study. Stroke 2004 Aug;35(8):1908-13. PMID: 15205487. **KQ3E6.**
186. Touvier M, Kesse E, Clavel-Chapelon F, et al. Dual Association of beta-carotene with risk of tobacco-related cancers in a cohort of French women. J Natl Cancer Inst 2005 Sep 21;97(18):1338-44. PMID: 16174855. **KQ3E5, KQ4E5.**
187. Varis K, Taylor PR, Sipponen P, et al. Gastric cancer and premalignant lesions in atrophic gastritis: a controlled trial on the effect of supplementation with alpha-tocopherol and beta-carotene. The Helsinki Gastritis Study Group. Scand J Gastroenterol 1998 Mar;33(3):294-300. PMID: 9548624. **KQ3E6.**
188. Vassilev ZP, Chu AF, Ruck B, et al. Evaluation of adverse drug reactions reported to a poison control center between 2000 and 2007. Am J Health Syst Pharm 2009;66(5 SUPPL. 3):X481-X487. PMID: 19233996. **KQ2E5, KQ4E5.**
189. Virtamo J, Edwards BK, Virtanen M, et al. Effects of supplemental alpha-tocopherol and beta-carotene on urinary tract cancer: incidence and mortality in a controlled trial (Finland). Cancer Causes Control 2000 Dec;11(10):933-9. PMID: 11142528. **KQ4E6.**
190. VITATOPS Trial Study Group, Hankey GJ, Algra A, et al. VITATOPS, the VITAmins TO prevent stroke trial: rationale and design of a randomised trial of B-vitamin therapy in patients with recent transient ischaemic attack or stroke (NCT00097669) (ISRCTN74743444). Int J Stroke 2007 May;2(2):144-50. PMID: 18705976. **KQ1E3.**
191. VITATOPS Trial Study Group. B vitamins in patients with recent transient ischaemic attack or stroke in the VITAmins TO Prevent Stroke (VITATOPS) trial: a randomised, double-blind, parallel, placebo-controlled trial. Lancet Neurology 2010 Sep;9(9):855-65. PMID: 20688574. **KQ1E3, KQ2E3.**
192. Walsh PC. Re: Vitamin e and the risk of prostate cancer: The Selenium and Vitamin e Cancer Prevention Trial (SELECT). J Urol 2012;187(5):1640-1. PMID: 22494720. **KQ4E6.**
193. Wang GQ, Dawsey SM, Li JY, et al. Effects of vitamin/mineral supplementation on the prevalence of histological dysplasia and early cancer of the esophagus and stomach: results from the General Population Trial in Linxian, China. Cancer Epidemiol Biomarkers Prev 1994 Mar;3(2):161-6. PMID: 8049638. **KQ1E2, KQ3E2.**
194. Wang L, Manson JE, Song Y, et al. Systematic review: Vitamin D and calcium supplementation in prevention of cardiovascular events. Ann Intern Med 2010 Mar 2;152(5):315-23. PMID: 20194238. **KQ3E9, KQ4E9.**
195. Wang X, Qin X, Demirtas H, et al. Efficacy of folic acid supplementation in stroke prevention: a meta-analysis. Lancet 2007 Jun 2;369(9576):1876-82. PMID: 17544768. **KQ3E3.**
196. Weingarten MA, Zalmanovici A, Yaphe J. Dietary calcium supplementation for preventing colorectal cancer and adenomatous polyps. Cochrane Database Syst Rev 2008(1):CD003548. PMID: 18254022. **KQ3E9.**
197. Wolf RL, Cauley JA, Pettinger M, et al. Lack of a relation between vitamin and mineral antioxidants and bone mineral density: results from the Women's Health Initiative. Am J Clin Nutr 2005 Sep;82(3):581-8. PMID: 16155271. **KQ3E6, KQ4E6.**

Appendix D. Excluded Studies

198. Wyatt G. Vitamin E increases prostate cancer risk in middle-aged men relative to placebo: no significant association observed with selenium, either alone or in combination with vitamin E. Evid Based Nurs 2012 Jul;15(3):90-1. PMID: 22411161. **KQ4E6.**
199. Xuan XZ, Schatzkin A, Mao BL, et al. Feasibility of conducting a lung-cancer chemoprevention trial among tin miners in Yunnan, P. R. China. Cancer Causes Control 1991 May;2(3):175-82. PMID: 1873448. **KQ2E3, KQ4E3.**
200. Zhang SM, Moore SC, Lin J, et al. Folate, vitamin B6, multivitamin supplements, and colorectal cancer risk in women. Am J Epidemiol 2006 Jan 15;163(2):108-15. PMID: 16339055. **KQ3E5, KQ4E5.**
201. Zhang SM, Cook NR, Albert CM, et al. Effect of combined folic acid, vitamin B6, and vitamin B12 on cancer risk in women: a randomized trial. JAMA 2008 Nov 5;300(17):2012-21. PMID: 18984888. **KQ1E3, KQ3E3, KQ4E3.**

Appendix E Table 1. Study Characteristics of Included Studies

Study Country USPSTF Quality	Study aim(s)	Study design	Inclusion criteria	Exclusion criteria	Intervention arm	N randomized
ACS[113,115,186] New Zealand Fair	Assess the long-term effects of calcium on bone density and fracture incidence; determine effect of calcium supplementation on CVD and death	RCT	Women age >55 years, >5 years postmenopausal, and life expectancy >5 years	Women receiving therapy for osteoporosis or taking calcium supplements; any other major ongoing disease, creatinine >1.8 mg/dL, untreated hypo- or hyperthyroidism, liver disease, serum 25-hydroxyvitamin D <10 mcg/L, malignancy, metabolic bone disease; regular users of HRT, anabolic steroids, glucocorticoids, or bisphosphonates in the previous year; lumbar spine bone density above the age-appropriate normal levels	Calcium 1,000 mg bid	732
					Placebo	739
AFPPS[101,102] United States and Canada Fair	Assess the safety and efficacy of folic acid supplementation for preventing colorectal cancer adenoma	RCT	Ages 21–80 years, had ≥1 of the following criteria: ≥1 histologically confirmed adenomas removed within 3 months before recruitment, ≥1 histologically confirmed adenomas removed within 16 months before recruitment, lifetime history of ≥2 confirmed adenomas, or a histologically confirmed adenoma of ≥1 cm in diameter before recruitment; complete colonoscopy with removal of all known polyps within 3 months of enrollment	History of familial polyposis syndromes, invasive large intestine cancer, malabsorption syndromes, any condition that could be worsened by supplemental aspirin or folic acid, or any condition commonly treated with aspirin, NSAIDs, or folate	Folic acid 1 mg qd	516
					Placebo	505
ASAP[79] Finland Fair	Determine efficacy of vitamin E and vitamin C supplementation on progression of carotid atherosclerosis	RCT, 2x2 factorial design*	Patients with hypercholesterolemia (serum cholesterol of ≥5.0 mmol/L) ages 45–69 years	Premenopausal, had regular oral estrogen substitution therapy, regular intake of antioxidants, ASA or any other drug with antioxidative properties, severely obese (BMI >32 kg/m^2), type 1 diabetes, uncontrolled hypertension (DBP >105 mm Hg), any condition limiting mobility making study visits impossible, severe disease-shortening life expectancy or other disease/condition worsening adherence to the measurements or treatment	Vitamin E 91 mg bid	130
					Vitamin C 250 mg bid	130
					Vitamin E 91 mg bid + vitamin C 250 mg bid	130
					Placebo	130

Appendix E Table 1. Study Characteristics of Included Studies

Study Country USPSTF Quality	Study aim(s)	Study design	Inclusion criteria	Exclusion criteria	Intervention arm	N randomized
ATBC[39,66,69-73,76-78,87,88,155-157] Finland Good	Reduce the incidence of lung cancer with vitamin E and/or beta-carotene supplementation; reduce the incidence of other cancer, CVD, and other chronic diseases	RCT, 2x2 factorial design	Male smokers (≥5 cigarettes per day) ages 50–69 years living in southwestern Finland	History of cancer (other than NMSC or CIS) or serious disease that would prevent (or limit) participation (severe angina on exertion [Rose criteria grade 2], chronic renal insufficiency, cirrhosis of liver, chronic alcoholism, psychiatric disorder, physical disability); taking supplements of vitamin E (>20 mg), vitamin A (>20,000 IU) or beta-carotene (>6 mg) in excess of predefined doses; treated with anticoagulants; nonsmokers	Vitamin E 50 mg qd	7,286
					Beta-carotene 20 mg qd	7,282
					Vitamin E 50 mg qd + beta-carotene 20 mg qd	7,278
					Placebo	7,287
CARET[60,67,74,161-164] United States Good	Determine the effect of beta-carotene plus vitamin A on preventing lung cancer in high-risk populations	RCT	Asbestos-exposed participants: men ages 45–69 years; exposed to asbestos on the job 15 years prior to randomization; chest x-ray positive for asbestos-related lung disease (fibrosis) or have worked in high-risk trades for 5 years; current smokers or have smoked in the last 15 years* Heavy smokers: men and women ages 50–69 years; had ≥20 pack-years smoking history; either currently smoking or had quit smoking within the previous 6 years†	NR	Beta-carotene 30 mg qd + vitamin A 25,000 IU qd	9,420
					Placebo	8,894
CPPS[114,116] United States Fair	Determine if calcium intake increases the risk of prostate cancer; impacts the recurrence of colorectal adenoma	RCT	Age <80 years; in good health; no history of familial polyposis, invasive large-bowel cancer, malabsorption syndromes, or any condition that might be worsened by supplemental calcium; men without a history of prostate cancer for prostate cancer publication only	NR	Calcium 1,200 mg bid	464
					Placebo	466

Appendix E Table 1. Study Characteristics of Included Studies

Study Country USPSTF Quality	Study aim(s)	Study design	Inclusion criteria	Exclusion criteria	Intervention arm	N randomized
Dean 2011[105] Australia Good	Assess whether vitamin D supplementation would lead to improvement in cognitive and emotional functioning	RCT	Healthy volunteers age ≥18 years with sufficient English language skills required to complete study protocol	Current use of vitamin D or calcium supplements; history of adverse reactions to vitamin supplements; current or past diagnosis of mood or psychotic disorder; history of neurologic illness, including cerebrovascular accident, CNS tumors head trauma, multiple sclerosis, epilepsy, movement disorder, or migraine treatment; current or recent (12 months) history of alcohol or illicit drug dependence; intellectual disability, pregnancy or currently breastfeeding or potential to become pregnant during the trial; history of severe renal impairment	Vitamin D 5,000 IU qd	63
					Placebo	65
Graat 2002[52] Netherlands Good	Determine if long-term supplementation of a multivitamin and/or vitamin E reduces the incidence and severity of acute respiratory tract infections	RCT, 2x2 factorial design*	Men and women age >60 years, noninstitutionalized	Used immunosuppressive treatment, anticoagulants interfering with vitamin K metabolism, dietary supplement in the previous 2 months or if they had a history of cancer, liver disease, or fat malabsorption during the 5 years prior to randomization	Multivitamin qd (vitamin A 600 mcg, beta-carotene 1.2 mg, vitamin C 60 mg, vitamin E 10 mg, vitamin D_3 5 mcg, vitamin K 30 mcg vitamin B_1 1.4 mg, vitamin B_2 1.6 mg, vitamin B_3 18 mg, vitamin B_5 6 mg, vitamin B_6 2 mg, biotin 150 mcg, folic acid 200 mcg, vitamin B_{12} 1 mcg, zinc 10 mg, selenium 25 mcg, iron 4 mg, Mg 30 mg, Cu 1 mg, iodine 100 mcg, calcium 74 mg, phosphor 49 mg, Mn 1 mg, Cr 25 mcg, Mo 25 mcg, silicium 2 mcg)	163
					Vitamin E 200 mg	164

Appendix E Table 1. Study Characteristics of Included Studies

Study Country USPSTF Quality	Study aim(s)	Study design	Inclusion criteria	Exclusion criteria	Intervention arm	N randomized
					Multivitamin qd (see above) + vitamin E 200 mg qd	172
					Placebo	153
IWHS[96] United States Good	Examine association between various lifestyle factors (e.g., supplement use) and morality, incidence of cancer, diabetes mellitus, hypertension, and fracture	Prospective cohort study	Women ages 55–69 years with a valid Iowa driver's license	Premenopausal at the time of the baseline questionnaire; had an implausible energy intake of <600 kcal or >5,000 kcal; failed to complete a substantial portion (>29 missing items) of the food frequency questionnaire; history of cancer other than skin cancer	Vitamin A†	12,293
					Nonusers of vitamin A	22,410
Lappe 2007[109,175] United States Fair	Determine the effect of calcium with or without vitamin D on skeletal status; determine efficacy in reducing incidence of cancer	RCT	Age >55 years, absence of known cancer, both mental and physical status sufficiently good to allow for 4-year participation in study; women only	NR	Calcium 1,400–1,500 mg qd§	445
					Calcium 1,400 mg qd + vitamin D_3 25 mcg qd	446
					Placebo	288
NHS[53] United States Good	Assess relationship between vitamin A supplementation and risk of hip fractures	Prospective cohort study	Postmenopausal (via natural or surgical menopause) registered nurses who responded to questionnaire in 1980	Previous hip fracture or diagnosis of cancer, heart disease, stroke, or osteoporosis	Supplement users (vitamin A, multivitamin, or beta-carotene)‡	NR
					Nonusers of supplements	NR
NPC[89,90,92-95,173] United States Fair	Determine if selenium supplementation reduces the incidence of BCC and SCC of the skin; reduces the incidence of other cancers	RCT	A history of ≥2 BCC or 1 SCC of the skin, with 1 of these occurring within the previous year; a 5-year life expectancy; no reported internal malignancies treated within the previous 5 years	History of significant kidney or liver disease	Selenium 200 mcg qd	653
					Brewer's yeast	659
NSCPS[84,160] Australia Good	Determine if beta-carotene can prevent skin cancer	RCT	Resident of Nambour, Queensland; ages 20–69 years when they took part in SCPS	Participants in prevalence study who were taking vitamin supplements containing beta-carotene and those already applying sunscreen on a strict daily basis were excluded	Beta-carotene 30 mg qd	820
					Placebo	801
PHS-I[51,55,58,158] United States Good	Assess the impact of beta-carotene supplementation on the incidence of cancer and CVD	RCT, 2x2 factorial design*§	U.S. male physicians; no history of cancer (except NMSC), MI, stroke, or transient cerebral ischema	History of the above conditions; current liver or renal disease, peptic ulcer, or gout; contraindications to aspirin consumption; current use of aspirin, other platelet-active drugs, or NSAIDs; current use of vitamin A supplement	Beta-carotene 50 mg qod	11,036
					No beta-carotene	11,035

Appendix E Table 1. Study Characteristics of Included Studies

Study Country USPSTF Quality	Study aim(s)	Study design	Inclusion criteria	Exclusion criteria	Intervention arm	N randomized
PHS-II (vitamin C and E arms)[80,83,154] United States Good	Evaluate whether long-term vitamin E or vitamin C supplementation decreases the risk of major cardiovascular events and cancer	RCT, 2x2x2 factorial design*‖	Male physicians age ≥55 years; men from PHS I with a history of MI, stroke, or cancer were eligible for PHS II (new participants were not eligible if they had a history of CVD or cancer)	Those unwilling to avoid using outside supplements; a history of cirrhosis or active liver disease in the past 6 months, cancer (except NMSC) (new participants), CVD (new participants), current renal disease, peptic ulcer, or gout; currently on anticoagulants	Vitamin E 400 IU qd	3,659
					Vitamin C 500 mg qd	3,673
					Vitamin E 400 IU qd + vitamin C 500 mg qd	3,656
					Placebo	3,653
PHS-II (multivitamin arm)[50] United States Good	Evaluate whether long-term multivitamin supplementation decreases the risk of major cardiovascular events and cancer	RCT, 2x2x2 factorial design*‖	Male physicians age ≥55 years; men from PHS I with a history of MI, stroke, or cancer were eligible for PHS II (new participants were not eligible if they had a history of CVD or cancer)	Those unwilling to avoid using outside supplements; a history of cirrhosis or active liver disease in the past 6 months, cancer (except NMSC) (new participants), CVD (new participants), current renal disease, peptic ulcer, or gout; currently on anticoagulants	Multivitamin	7,317
					Placebo	7,324
REACT[51] United States and United Kingdom Good	Determine if multivitamin use would impact the progression of age-related cataracts	RCT	Age ≥40 years; ≥1 eyes met the following criteria: cataract extraction unlikely within 2 years, immature idiopathic "senile" cataract present, presence of minimal cataract by Lens Opacities Classification System criteria (U.S. patients), presence of cataract of minimal Oxford grade (U.K. patients), LogMAR acuity ≤0.5, no clinical signs of glaucoma and intraocular pressure by applanation tonometry ≤25 mm HG; no history of amblyopia, eye surgery, argon or YAG laser treatment, or major eye trauma; no history of iritis, renal crystalline deposits, or optic nerve disease; no extended use of ocular corticosteroid or glaucoma therapy; no participation in another clinical trial investigating an anticataract formulation within the last year	Pregnant; history of diabetes mellitus, severe renal failure, or kidney stones, fat malabsorption syndrome, major intestinal surgery, chronic diarrhea, alcoholism, extended use of corticosteroid treatment, use of anticoagulants, regular use of any vitamin supplement	Multivitamin tid (vitamin C 250 mg, vitamin E 200 mg, and beta-carotene 6 mg)	149
					Placebo	148

Appendix E Table 1. Study Characteristics of Included Studies

Study Country USPSTF Quality	Study aim(s)	Study design	Inclusion criteria	Exclusion criteria	Intervention arm	N randomized
RECORD[103,107] United Kingdom Fair	Investigate whether vitamin D or calcium supplementation affects mortality, vascular disease, and cancer in older people	RCT, 2x2 factorial design*	Older adults age ≥70 years with a fragility fracture	Cancer likely to metastasize to bone within the previous 10 years; bed- or chairbound before fracture, Abbreviated Mental Test score <7, fracture associated with preexisting local bone abnormality, known hypercalcemia, renal stone in the last 10 years, life expectancy <6 months, known to be leaving the United Kingdom, taking >200 IU (5 μg) of vitamin D or >500 mg calcium supplements daily, treatment with fluoride, bisphosphonates, calcitonin, tibolone, HRT, SERMs, or any vitamin D metabolite (e.g., calcitriol) in the last 5 years or vitamin D by injection in the last year	Calcium 1,000 mg qd	1,311
					Vitamin D$_3$ 800 IU qd	1,343
					Calcium 1,000 mg qd + vitamin D 800 IU qd	1,306
					Placebo	1,332
SCPS[63,75,159] United States Fair	Determine if beta-carotene supplementation increases the time to occurrence of first skin cancer	RCT	≥1 biopsy-proven BCC or SCC since January 1, 1980; age <85 years; no potential childbearing; agree not to take vitamin supplements containing vitamin A or beta-carotene; not a vegan vegetarian	Active cancer other than skin cancer; xeroderma pigmentosum; basal cell nevus syndrome; significant known arsenic exposure; other major medical problems that might limit participation (e.g., disabling CVD, active liver disease, alcohol or drug dependence)	Beta-carotene 50 mg qd	913
					Placebo	892
SELECT[82,143,166-169] United States, Canada, and Puerto Rico Good	Reduce the risk of prostate cancer with selenium and/or vitamin E, as well as other cancers and cardiovascular events	RCT, 2x2 factorial deign	Healthy men age ≥50 years (African American) or ≥55 years (all other races); normal blood pressure; serum PSA ≥4 ng/mL; DRE not suspicious for cancer; willing to restrict off-study supplement use; SWOG performance status = 0.	Prior history of prostate cancer or high-grade prostatic intraepithelial neoplasia; anticoagulation therapy other than ≥175 mg/day ASA or ≥81 mg/day ASA with clopidogrel bisulfate; history of hemorrhagic stroke	Vitamin E 400 IU qd	8,904
					Selenium 200 mcg qd	8,910
					Vitamin E 400 IU qd + selenium 200 mcg qd	8,863
					Placebo	8,856

Appendix E Table 1. Study Characteristics of Included Studies

Study Country USPSTF Quality	Study aim(s)	Study design	Inclusion criteria	Exclusion criteria	Intervention arm	N randomized
SKICAPS-AK[97,174] United States Fair	Determine the efficacy of vitamin A supplementation on the incidence of first NMSC in moderate-risk patients	RCT	Ages 21–85 years; ambulatory and capable of self-care; no diagnosis of life-threatening condition or internal cancer in past year; normal or near normal laboratory values in a routine screening panel of tests; planning to live within travel distance of SKICAP clinic for ≥5 years; willing to limit nonstudy vitamin A supplementation to ≤10,000 IU/day; history of ≥10 pathologically confirmed actinic keratoses (most recent diagnosed within preceding year) and a pathologically confirmed record of ≤1 prior SCC or BCC	NR	Vitamin A 25,000 IU qd Placebo	1,157 1,140
SKICAPS-S/B[98,174] United States Fair	Determine the effect of vitamin A and isotretinoin on the incidence of NMSC in high-risk patients	RCT	Ages 21–85 years; ambulatory and capable of self-care; no diagnosis of life-threatening condition or internal cancer in past year; normal or near normal laboratory values in a routine screening panel of tests; planning to live within travel distance of SKICAP clinic for ≥5 years; history of ≥4 pathologically confirmed BCC or cutaneous SCC; triglyceride level <95% UL of normal; no childbearing potential or breastfeeding	Patients with a diagnosis of basal cell nevus syndrome or xeroderma pigmentosum	Vitamin A 25,000 IU qd Placebo	173 174
SU.VI.MAX[49,54,56,58,151-153] France Good	Reduce the incidence of cancer and ischemic heart disease with multivitamin supplementation	RCT	Men (ages 45–60 years) and women (ages 35–60 years), free of any severe pathology that might limit participation, not be taking supplements containing any of the study vitamins or minerals, express no ambiguous motivations or	NR	Multivitamin qd (vitamin C 120 mg, vitamin E 30 mg, beta-carotene 6 mg, selenium 100 mcg, and zinc 20 mg)	6,481

Appendix E Table 1. Study Characteristics of Included Studies

Study Country USPSTF Quality	Study aim(s)	Study design	Inclusion criteria	Exclusion criteria	Intervention arm	N randomized
			obsessional behavior concerning diet and health; manifest no qualms about complying with protocol constraints		Placebo	6,536
Trivedi 2003[104] United Kingdom Fair	Determine the effect of vitamin D supplementation on rate of fractures	RCT	Men and women ages 65–85 years	Already taking vitamin D supplements, conditions that were contraindications to vitamin D supplements (e.g., renal stones, sarcoidosis, or malignancy)	Vitamin D_3 100,000 IU every 4 months	1,345
					Placebo	1,341
U.K. PRECISE[91] United Kingdom Fair	Determine the effect of selenium supplementation on cancer prevention	RCT	Elderly volunteers ages 60–74 years	SWOG score >1, active liver or kidney disease, prior diagnosis of cancer (excluding NMSC), diagnosed HIV infection, immunosuppressive therapy, diminished mental capacity, taking ≥50 mcg/d of selenium supplements in the previous 6 months	Selenium 100 mcg qd	127
					Selenium 200 mcg qd	127
					Selenium 300 mcg qd	126
					Placebo	121
WHI[108,110,111,137,176-184] United States Good	Evaluate the efficacy of calcium with vitamin D supplementation on preventing colorectal cancer; evaluate the efficacy of preventing hip and other fractures	RCT	Participants enrolled in the WHI dietary modification trial, hormone therapy trials, or both; women ages 50–79 years at initial screening; no evidence of a medical condition associated with a predicted survival of <3 years; no safety, adherence, or retention risks	Hypercalcemia; renal calculi; corticosteroid or calcitriol use; intention to continue to take ≥600 IU of vitamin D per day of personal supplements	Vitamin D_3 200 IU bid + calcium 500 mg bid	18,176
					Placebo	18,106
WHS[62,81,185] United States Good	Prevent cancer and CVD with vitamin E or beta-carotene supplementation	RCT, 2x2x2 factorial design¶	Women age ≥45 years; postmenopausal or had no intention of becoming pregnant; no previous history of CHD, cerebrovascular disease, cancer (except NMSC), or any serious illness that might preclude participation; no reported history of serious side effects to any study treatment; not currently taking ASA, ASA-containing medications, or NSAIDs ≥1/week or willing to forgo the use of these; not currently taking anticoagulants or corticosteroids; and not taking vitamin A or E or beta-carotene supplements >1/week	Participants in the ongoing Nurses' Health Study (an observational cohort study of registered nurses)	Vitamin E 600 IU qod	19,937
					No vitamin E	19,939
					Beta-carotene 50 mg qod	19,939
					No beta-carotene	19,937

Appendix E Table 1. Study Characteristics of Included Studies

*Factorial design studies may have reported outcomes by original randomized arms and/or by factorial design; i.e., participants who were randomized to receive a specific supplement (e.g., vitamin C with or without vitamin E) vs. participants not randomized to receive the aforementioned specific supplement (e.g., vitamin E alone or placebo).

†IWHS: prospective cohort study among women taking vitamin A compared with nonusers of vitamin A; dosage not reported.

‡NHS: prospective cohort study among women taking one of the following supplements: multivitamin, vitamin A, or beta-carotene compared with nonusers; dosage or number of participants by supplement not reported.

§PHS-I: participants randomized to receive beta-carotene, beta-carotene + aspirin, aspirin, or placebo; numbers of participants allocated to original randomized arms not reported.

‖PHS-II: participants randomized to receive vitamin E, vitamin C, multivitamin, beta-carotene (discontinued), or placebo.

¶WHS: participants randomized to receive vitamin E, beta-carotene, aspirin, or placebo; numbers of participants allocated to original randomized arms not reported.

Abbreviations: ACS = Auckland Calcium Study; AFPPS = Aspirin/Folate Polyp Prevention Study; ASA = acetylsalicylic acid; ASAP = Antioxidant Supplementation in Atherosclerosis Prevention; ATBC = Alpha-Tocopherol Beta-Carotene Cancer Prevention; bid = twice daily; BCC = basal cell carcinoma; BMI = body mass index; CARET = Carotene and Retinol Efficacy Trial; CHD = coronary heart disease; CIS = carcinoma in situ; CNS = central nervous system; CPPS = Calcium Polyp Prevention Study; CVD = cardiovascular disease; DBP = diastolic blood pressure; DRE = digital rectal examination; HRT = hormone replacement therapy; IWHS = Iowa Women's Health Study; LogMAR = logarithm of the minimum angle of resolution; MI = myocardial infarction; NHS = Nurses' Health Study; NMSC = nonmelanoma skin cancer; NPC = Nutritional Prevention of Cancer; NR = not reported; NSAID = nonsteroidal anti-inflammatory drug; NSCPS = Nambour Skin Cancer Prevention Study; PHS = Physician's Health Study; PSA = prostate-specific antigen; qd = once daily; qod = every other day; RCT = randomized, controlled trial; REACT = Roche European American Cataract Trial; RECORD = Randomized Evaluation of Calcium or Vitamin D; SCC = squamous cell carcinoma; SCPS = Skin Cancer Prevention Study; SELECT = Selenium and Vitamin E Cancer Prevention Trial; SERM = selective estrogen receptor modulator; SKICAP-AK = Skin Cancer Prevention Trial-Actinic Keratoses; SKICAP=S/B = Skin Cancer Prevention Trial-SCC/BCC; SU.VI.MAX = Supplementation in Vitamins and Mineral Antioxidants Study; SWOG = Southwest Oncology Group; U.K. PRECISE = U.K. Prevention of Cancer by Intervention with Selenium; UL = upper intake limit; WHI = Women's Health Initiative; WHS = Women's Health Study; YAG = yttrium aluminium garnet.

Appendix E Table 2. Baseline Demographics of Included Studies (Entire Study Population)

Study	Supplement(s)	N randomized	Mean age (years)	Female (%)	Nonwhite (%)	Mean BMI (kg/m^2)	Current smokers (%)	Alcohol use	Prior supplement use (%)
ACS[13,115,186]	Calcium	1,471	74.3	100	NR	26.4	3.0	NR	NR
AFPPS[101,102]	Folic acid	1,021	57	36.3	14.4	27.4	14.4	0.6 drinks/day	MVI: 35.9
ASAP[79]	Vitamin E, vitamin C	520	59.8	51	NR	NR	40.4	58.6 g/week	NR
ATBC[59,66,69-73,76-78,87,88,155-157]	Beta-carotene, vitamin E	29,133	57.2	0	NR	26.3	100	18.0 g/day	NR
CARET[60,67,74,161-164]	Beta-carotene + vitamin A	18,314	57.5	34.3	6.8	NR	60.1	NR	NR
CPPS[114,116]	Calcium	930	61.9	28	5.4 (men only)	NR	NR	NR	Calcium: 3
Dean 2011[105]	Vitamin D	128	21.8	57	NR	NR	NR	NR	NR
Graat 2002[52]	Multivitamin, vitamin E	652	73.2	50	NR	27.4	9	NR	39
IWHS[95]	Vitamin A	34,703	61	100	0.7	27.0	NR	3.8 g/day	Vitamin A: 35
Lappe 2007[109,175]	Calcium, vitamin D	1,180	66.7	100	0	29.0	NR	NR	NR
NHS[53]	Multivitamin, vitamin A, beta-carotene	72,337	58.3	100	NR	26.0	26	7.4 g/day	MVI: 17 Vitamin A: 0.6 Beta-carotene: 0.8
NPC[89,90,92-95,172,173]	Selenium	1,312	63	0	NR	26	28	NR	NR
NSCPS[84,160]	Beta-carotene	1,621	48.7	56	NR	NR	NR	NR	NR
PHS-I[81,55,88,158]	Beta-carotene	22,071	NR	0	NR	NR	11	NR	MVI: 20
PHS-II[50,57,80,83,154]	Vitamin E, vitamin C, multivitamin	14,641	64.3	0	NR	26.0	3.6	80.7% consume ≥1 drink/month	NR
REACT[51]	Multivitamin	297	66.2	59.3	NR	NR	18.8	NR	0
RECORD[103,107]	Calcium, vitamin D	5,292	77	84.7	0.8	NR	11.7	NR	NR
SCPS[63,75,159]	Beta-carotene	1,805	63.0	30.7	NR	NR	18.7	NR	Daily: 23.9 Occasionally: 15.6
SELECT[82,143,165-169]	Vitamin E, selenium	35,533	62.5	0	21	NR	8	NR	NR
SKICAP-AK[97,174]	Vitamin A	2,297	63	30	NR	NR	12	NR	Sometimes: 28.5 Yes: 44.5
SKICAP-SB[98,174]	Vitamin A	347	NR	28	NR	NR	NR	NR	Sometimes: 27 Yes: 47.5
SU.VI.MAX[49,54-56,58,151-153]	Multivitamin	13,017	49.0	59.0	NR	NR	15.9	NR	NR
Trivedi 2003[104]	Vitamin D, calcium	2,686	74.8	24.2	NR	24.3	4.2	71.7% regular users	Vitamin D: 0
UK PRECISE[91]	Selenium	501	67.5	47.4	NR	24.4	9.5	86.9% current users	NR
WHI[108,110,111,137,176-184]	Vitamin D + calcium	36,282	62.4	100	16.9	27.5	7.6	71.3% current users	Calcium: 29.0 MVI: 36.7

Appendix E Table 2. Baseline Demographics of Included Studies (Entire Study Population)

Study	Supplement(s)	N randomized	Mean age (years)	Female (%)	Nonwhite (%)	Mean BMI (kg/m^2)	Current smokers (%)	Alcohol use	Prior supplement use (%)
WHS[52,81,165]	Vitamin E, beta-carotene	39,876	54.6	100	NR	26.0	13.1	54.9% consume alcohol ≥1/month	MVI: 38.8

Abbreviations: ACS = Auckland Calcium Study; AFPPS = Aspirin/Folate Polyp Prevention Study; ASAP = Antioxidant Supplementation in Atherosclerosis Prevention; ATBC = Alpha-Tocopherol Beta-Carotene Cancer Prevention; BMI = body mass index; CARET = Carotene and Retinol Efficacy Trial; CPPS = Calcium Polyp Prevention Study; IWHS = Iowa Women's Health Study; MVI = multivitamin; NHS = Nurses' Health Study; NPC = Nutritional Prevention of Cancer; NR = not reported; NSCPS = Nambour Skin Cancer Prevention Study; PHS = Physician's Health Study; REACT = Roche European American Cataract Trial; RECORD = Randomized Evaluation of Calcium or Vitamin D; SCPS = Skin Cancer Prevention Study; SELECT = Selenium and Vitamin E Cancer Prevention Trial; SKICAP-AK = Skin Cancer Prevention Trial-Actinic Keratoses; SKICAP=S/B = Skin Cancer Prevention Trial-SCC/BCC; SU.VI.MAX = Supplementation in Vitamins and Mineral Antioxidants Study; U.K. PRECISE = U.K. Prevention of Cancer by Intervention with Selenium; WHI = Women's Health Initiative; WHS = Women's Health Study.

Appendix F Table 1. Cancer Incidence, Cancer Mortality, and All-Cause Mortality Among Beta-Carotene Alone vs. Placebo Arms of ATBC Trial[73,76,77]

Outcome	Mean followup (y)	Intervention, # of subjects with events (%)	Comparator, # of subjects with events (%)	RR	95% CI	P-value
Lung cancer*	8	242/7,282 (3.3)	209/7,287 (2.9)	1.16	0.97 to 1.40	NR
	11	140/6,281 (2.2)	120/6,375 (1.9)	1.19	0.93 to 1.52	NR
	14	120/5,625 (2.1)	130/5,782 (2.2)	0.97	0.76 to 1.25	NR
Prostate cancer*†	6.1	80/7,282 (1.1)	67/7,287 (0.9)	1.20	0.87 to 1.66	NR
	8	82/7,282 (1.1)	67/7,287 (0.9)	1.23	0.89 to 1.70	NR
	11	73/6,306 (1.2)	74/6,388 (1.2)	1.00	0.73 to 1.39	NR
	14	106/5,615 (1.9)	104/5,745 (1.8)	1.05	0.80 to 1.38	NR
Colorectal cancer*†‡	6.1	39/7,282 (0.5)	37/7,287 (0.5)	1.06	0.68 to 1.66	NR
	8	39/7,282 (0.5)	37/7,287 (0.5)	1.06	0.67 to 1.66	NR
	11	22/6,340 (0.3)	20/6,416 (0.3)	1.12	0.61 to 2.05	NR
	14	38/5,677 (0.7)	18/5,806 (0.3)	2.18	1.25 to 3.82	NR
Colorectal cancer death	6.1	13/7,282 (0.2)	11/7,287 (0.2)	NR	NR	NR
Prostate cancer death	6.1	21/7,282 (0.3)	18/7,287 (0.2)	NR	NR	NR
All-cause mortality	8	919/7,282 (12.6)	851/7,287 (11.7)	1.08	0.99 to 1.19	NR
	11	651/6,363 (10.2)	598/6,436 (9.3)	1.11	0.99 to 1.24	NR
	14	728/5,712 (12.7)	668/5,838 (11.4)	1.12	1.01 to 1.25	NR
	16	495/4,984 (9.9)	488/5,170 (9.4)	1.06	0.93 to 1.20	NR

*Overall 6-year posttrial followup: lung cancer RR, 1.06 (95% CI, 0.94 to 1.20); prostate cancer RR 1.06 (95% CI, 0.91 to 1.23), colorectal cancer RR, 1.44 (95% CI, 1.09 to 1.90).
†Subsequent ATBC publications after the initial publication[59] reclassified cancer cases: three additional prostate cancer cases were identified and seven were reclassified as nonmalignant; colorectal cancer cases excluded six participants with carcinoids and squamous cell carcinoma of the anal canal, an additional eight colorectal cancer cases were reclassified based on pathology.
‡Combined colon and rectal cancer cases.

Abbreviations: ATBC = Alpha-Tocopherol Beta-Carotene Cancer Prevention; CI = confidence interval; NR = not reported; RR = relative risk; y = years.

Appendix F Table 2. Cancer Incidence, Cancer Mortality, and All-Cause Mortality Among Vitamin E Alone vs. Placebo Arms of the ATBC Trial[73,76,77]

Outcome	Mean followup (y)	Intervention, # of subjects with events (%)	Comparator, # of subjects with events (%)	RR	95% CI	P-value
Lung cancer	11	205/7,286 (2.8)	209/7,287 (2.9)	0.98	0.81 to 1.19	NR
	14	112/6,349 (1.8)	120/6,375 (1.9)	0.94	0.73 to 1.21	NR
	16	147/5,780 (2.5)	130/5,782 (2.2)	1.14	0.90 to 1.44	NR
Prostate cancer	6.1–11	43/7,286 (0.6)	67/7,287 (0.9)	0.64	0.44 to 0.94	NR
	14	54/6,349 (0.9)	74/6,375 (1.2)	0.73	0.51 to 1.04	NR
	16	98/5,780 (1.7)	104/5,782 (1.8)	0.94	0.72 to 1.24	NR
Colorectal cancer	6.1	29/7,286 (0.4)	37/7,287 (0.5)	0.79	0.48 to 1.28	NR
	11	29/7,286 (0.4)	37/7,287 (0.5)	0.78	0.48 to 1.28	NR
	14	25/6,349 (0.4)	20/6,375 (0.3)	1.25	0.70 to 2.26	NR
	16	22/5,780 (0.4)	18/5,782 (0.3)	1.23	0.66 to 2.29	NR
Prostate cancer death	11	11/7,286 (0.2)	18/7,287 (0.2)	NR	NR	NR
Colorectal cancer death	6.1	12/7,286 (0.2)	11/7,287 (0.2)	NR	NR	NR
All-cause mortality	8	868/7,286 (11.9)	851/7,287 (11.7)	1.02	0.93 to 1.12	NR
	11	566/6,349 (8.9)	598/6,375 (9.4)	0.95	0.85 to 1.07	NR
	14	733/5,780 (12.7)	668/5,782 (11.6)	1.10	0.99 to 1.23	NR
	16	504/5,119 (9.8)	488/5,170 (9.4)	1.05	0.93 to 1.19	NR

Abbreviations: ATBC = Alpha-Tocopherol Beta-Carotene Cancer Prevention; CI = confidence interval; NR = not reported; RR = relative risk.

Appendix F Table 3. Cancer Incidence, Cancer Mortality, and All-Cause Mortality Among Beta-Carotene Combined With Vitamin E vs. Placebo Arms of the ATBC Trial[73,76,77]

Outcome	Mean followup (m)	Intervention, # of subjects (%)	Comparator, # of subjects (%)	RR†	95% CI	P-value
Lung cancer	96	239/7,278 (3.3)	209/7,287 (2.9)	1.15	0.96 to 1.38	NR
	132*	126/6,278 (2)	120/6,375 (1.9)	1.07	0.83 to 1.38	NR
	168*	140/5,651 (2.5)	130/5,782 (2.2)	1.11	0.87 to 1.41	NR
Prostate cancer	73.2	56/7,278 (0.8)	67/7,287 (0.9)	1.23‡	0.96 to 1.58	0.088
	96	56/7,278 (0.8)	67/7,287 (0.9)	0.84	0.59 to 1.20	NR
	132*	76/6,308 (1.2)	74/6,388 (1.2)	1.05	0.76 to 1.44	NR
	168*	87/5,622 (1.5)	104/5,745 (1.8)	0.86	0.65 to 1.15	NR
Colorectal cancer	73.2	30/7,278 (0.4)	37/7,287 (0.5)	0.82	0.50 to 1.32	NR
	96	30/7,278 (0.4)	37/7,287 (0.5)	0.81	0.50 to 1.32	NR
	132*	25/6,330 (0.4)	20/6,416 (0.3)	1.27	0.71 to 2.29	NR
	168*	35/5,696 (0.6)	18/5,806 (0.3)	2.00	1.13 to 3.54	NR
Prostate cancer death	73.2	12/7,278 (0.2)	18/7,287 (0.2)	NR	NR	NR
Colorectal cancer death	73.2	10/7,278 (0.1)	11/7,287 (0.2)	NR	NR	NR
All-cause mortality	96	932/7,278 (12.8)	851/7,287 (11.7)	1.10	1.00 to 1.21	NR
	132*	627/6,346 (9.9)	598/6,436 (9.3)	1.07	0.96 to 1.20	NR
	168*	727/5,719 (12.7)	668/5,838 (11.4)	1.12	1.01 to 1.25	NR
	192*	476/4,992 (9.5)	488/5,170 (9.4)	1.01	0.89 to 1.15	NR

*Posttrial followup 3 and 6 years after end of intervention.
†Crude RR reported unless otherwise specified.
‡Adjusted for age, number of cigarettes, years of smoking, and fat intake.

Abbreviations: ATBC = Alpha-Tocopherol Beta-Carotene Cancer Prevention; CI = confidence interval; m = month; NR = not reported; RR = relative risk.

Appendix F Table 4. Cardiovascular Disease and Cancer Incidence, Mortality, and All-Cause Mortality Among Vitamin D Alone vs. Placebo Arms of the RECORD Trial[103]

Outcome	Mean followup (y)	Intervention, # of subjects (%)	Comparator, # of subjects (%)	RR	95% CI	P-value
Any CVD death	6.2	173/1,343 (12.9)	182/1,332 (13.7)	NR	NR	NR
Fatal CHD	6.2	74/1,343 (5.5)	85/1,332 (6.4)	NR	NR	NR
Fatal stroke	6.2	59/1,343 (4.4)	51/1,332 (3.8)	NR	NR	NR
Any cancer	6.2	187/1,343 (13.9)	165/1,332 (12.4)	NR	NR	NR
Breast cancer	6.2	23/1,343 (1.7)	16/1,332 (1.2)	NR	NR	NR
Colorectal cancer	6.2	17/1,343 (1.3)	8/1,332 (0.6)	NR	NR	NR
Lung cancer	6.2	14/1,343 (1.0)	18/1,332 (1.4)	NR	NR	NR
Prostate cancer	6.2	9/1,343 (0.7)	8/1,332 (0.6)	NR	NR	NR
Any cancer death	6.2	73/1,343 (5.4)	78/1,332 (5.9)	NR	NR	NR
Breast cancer death	6.2	7/1,343 (0.5)	4/1,332 (0.3)	NR	NR	NR
Colorectal cancer death	6.2	7/1,343 (0.5)	6/1,332 (0.5)	NR	NR	NR
Lung cancer death	6.2	10/1,343 (0.7)	21/1,332 (1.6)	NR	NR	NR
All-cause mortality	6.2	421/1,343 (31.3)	434/1,332 (32.6)	NR	NR	NR

Abbreviations: CHD = coronary heart disease; CI = confidence interval; CVD = cardiovascular disease; NR = not reported; RECORD = Randomized Evaluation of Calcium or Vitamin D; RR = relative risk; y = years.

Appendix F Table 5. Cardiovascular Disease and Cancer Incidence, Mortality, and All-Cause Mortality Among Calcium Alone vs. Placebo Arms of the RECORD Trial[103]

Outcome	Mean followup (y)	Intervention, # of subjects (%)	Comparator, # of subjects (%)	RR	95% CI	P-value
Any CVD death	6.2	194/1,311 (14.8)	182/1,332 (13.7)	NR	NR	NR
Fatal stroke	6.2	54/1,311 (4.1)	51/1,332 (3.8)	NR	NR	NR
Fatal vascular disease	6.2	91/1,311 (6.9)	85/1,332 (6.4)	NR	NR	NR
Any cancer	6.2	189/1,311 (14.4)	165/1,332 (12.4)	NR	NR	NR
Breast cancer	6.2	21/1,311 (1.6)	16/1,332 (1.2)	NR	NR	NR
Colorectal cancer	6.2	22/1,311 (1.7)	8/1,332 (0.6)	NR	NR	NR
Lung cancer	6.2	14/1,311 (1.1)	18/1,332 (1.3)	NR	NR	NR
Prostate cancer	6.2	4/1,311 (0.3)	8/1,332 (0.6)	NR	NR	NR
Any cancer death	6.2	95/1,311 (7.2)	78/1,332 (5.9)	NR	NR	NR
Breast cancer death	6.2	9/1,311 (.6)	4/1,332 (.3)	NR	NR	NR
Colorectal cancer death	6.2	7/1,311 (0.5)	6/1,332 (0.5)	NR	NR	NR
Lung cancer death	6.2	13/1,311 (1)	21/1,332 (1.6)	NR	NR	NR
Prostate cancer death	6.2	3/1,311 (0.2)	3/1,332 (0.2)	NR	NR	NR
All-cause mortality	6.2	447/1,311 (34.1)	434/1,332 (32.6)	NR	NR	NR

Abbreviations: CI = confidence interval; CVD = cardiovascular disease; NR = not reported; RECORD = Randomized Evaluation of Calcium or Vitamin D; RR = relative risk; y = years.

Appendix F Table 6. Cardiovascular Disease and Cancer Incidence, Mortality, and All-Cause Mortality Among Vitamin D Combined With Calcium vs. Placebo Arms of the RECORD Trial[103]

Outcome	Mean followup (y)	Intervention, # of subjects (%)	Comparator, # of subjects (%)	RR	95% CI	P-value
Any CVD death	6.2	177/1,306 (13.6)	182/1,332 (13.6)	NR	NR	NR
Fatal stroke	6.2	56/1,306 (4.3)	51/1,332 (3.8)	NR	NR	NR
Fatal CHD	6.2	88/1,306 (6.7)	85/1,332 (6.4)	NR	NR	NR
Any cancer	6.2	182/1,306 (13.9)	165/1,332 (12.4)	NR	NR	NR
Breast cancer	6.2	20/1,306 (1.5)	16/1,332 (1.2)	NR	NR	NR
Colorectal cancer	6.2	24/1,306 (1.8)	8/1,332 (0.6)	NR	NR	NR
Lung cancer	6.2	10/1,306 (0.8)	18/1,332 (1.4)	NR	NR	NR
Prostate cancer	6.2	8/1,306 (0.6)	17/1,332 (1.3)	NR	NR	NR
Any cancer death	6.2	83/1,306 (6.4)	78/1,332 (5.9)	NR	NR	NR
Breast cancer death	6.2	7/1,306 (0.5)	4/1,332 (0.3)	NR	NR	NR
Colorectal cancer death	6.2	13/1,306 (1.0)	6/1,332 (0.5)	NR	NR	NR
Lung cancer death	6.2	14/1,306 (1.1)	21/1,332 (1.6)	NR	NR	NR
Prostate cancer death	6.2	2/1,306 (0.2)	3/1,332 (0.2)	NR	NR	NR
All-cause mortality	6.2	415/1,306 (31.8)	434/1,336 (32.5)	NR	NR	NR

Abbreviations: CHD = coronary heart disease; CI = confidence interval; CVD = cardiovascular disease; NR = not reported; RECORD = Randomized Evaluation of Calcium or Vitamin D; RR = relative risk; y = years.

Appendix F Figure 1. Relative Risk for Any Cancer Incidence at Longest Followup Only, by Supplement, Original Randomized Arms of the RECORD Trial

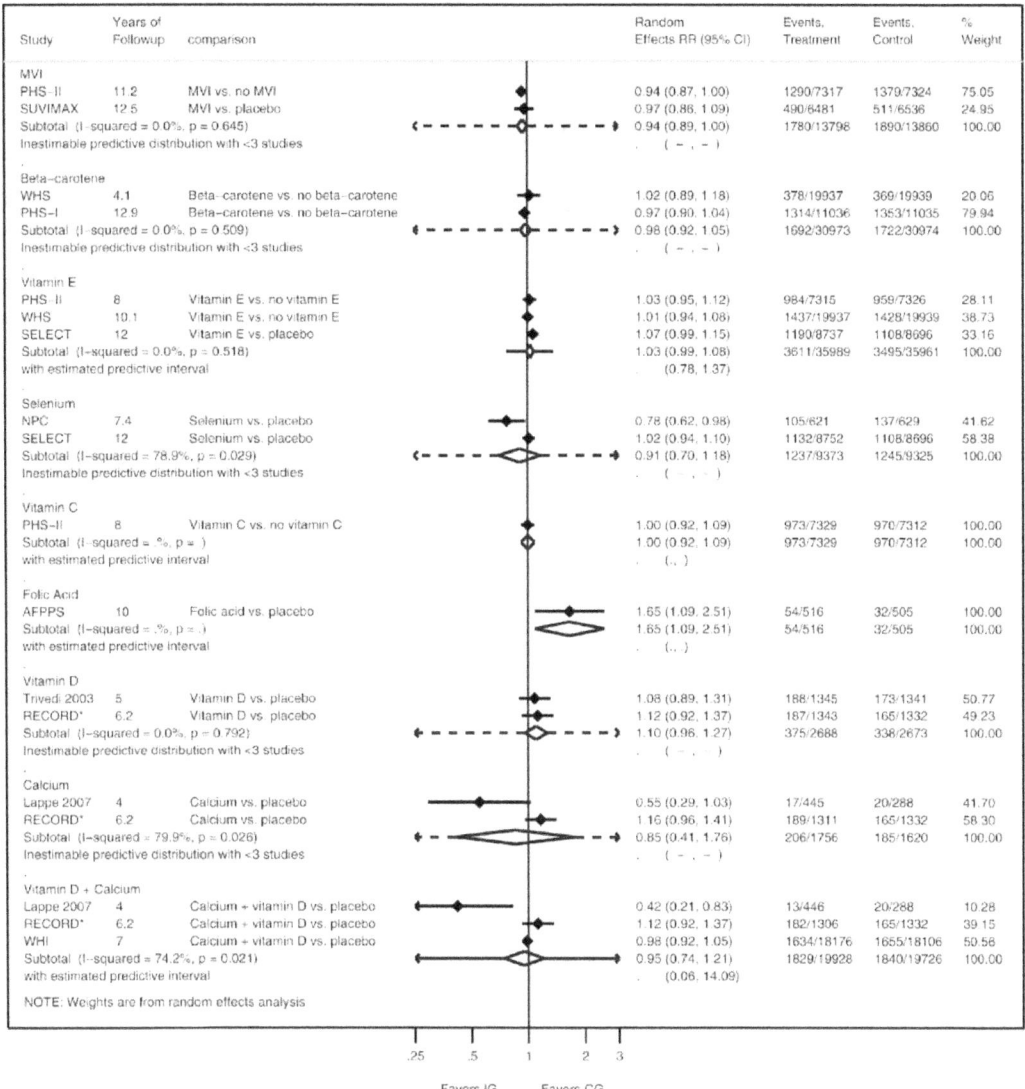

Abbreviations: AFPPS = Aspirin/Folate Polyp Prevention Study; CG = control group; CI = confidence interval; IG = intervention group; MVI = multivitamin; NPC = Nutritional Prevention of Cancer; PHS = Physician's Health Study; RECORD = Randomized Evaluation of Calcium or Vitamin D; RR = relative risk; SELECT = Selenium and Vitamin E Cancer Prevention Trial; SU.VI.MAX = Supplementation in Vitamins and Mineral Antioxidants Study; WHI = Women's Health Initiative; WHS = Women's Health Study.

Appendix F Figure 2. Relative Risk for All-Cause Mortality at Longest Followup Only, by Supplement, Original Randomized Arms of the RECORD Trial

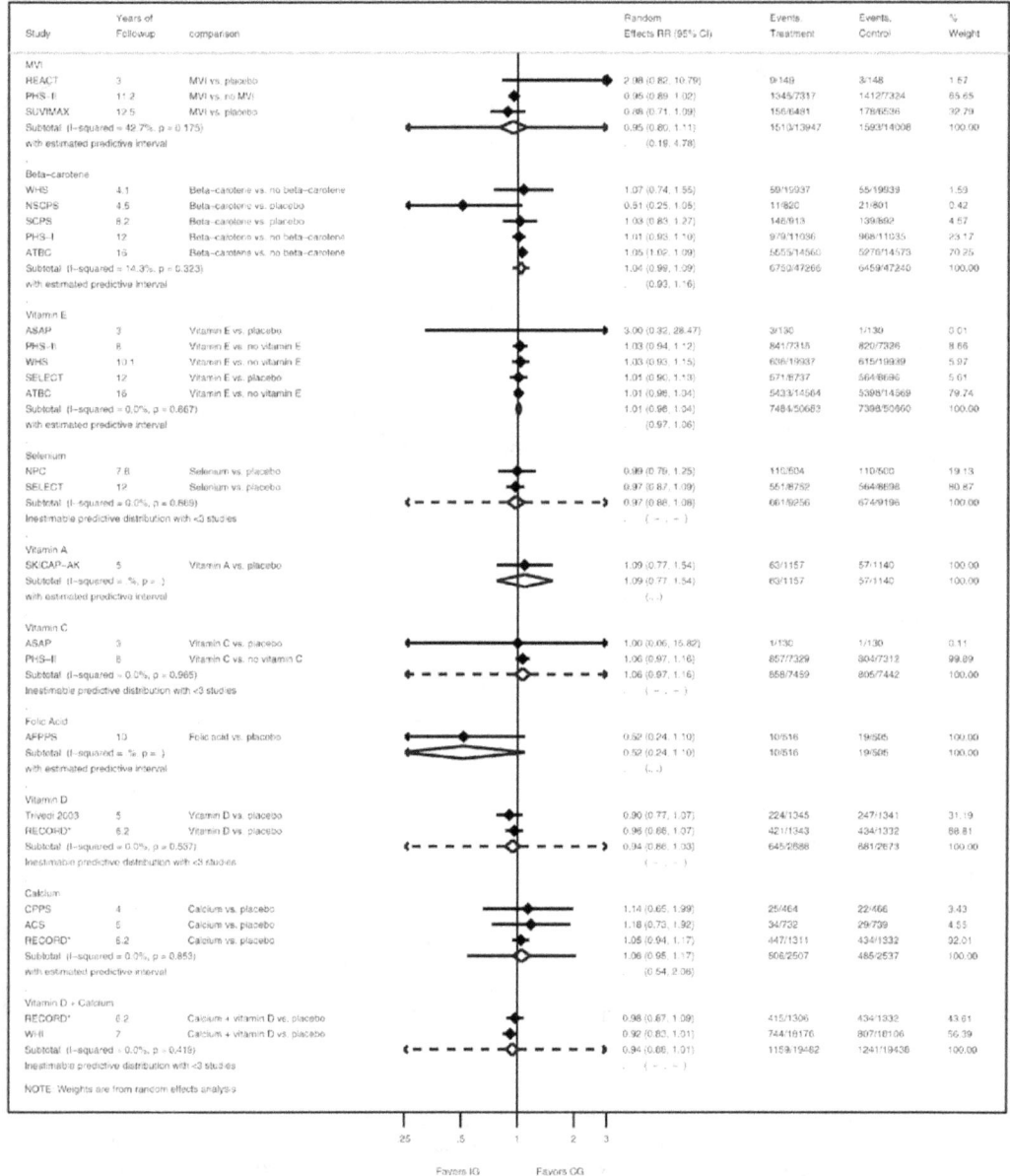

Abbreviations: ACS = Auckland Calcium Study; AFPPS = Aspirin/Folate Polyp Prevention Study; ASAP = Antioxidant Supplementation in Atherosclerosis Prevention; ATBC = Alpha-Tocopherol Beta-Carotene Cancer Prevention; CI = confidence interval; CPPS = Calcium Polyp Prevention Study; MVI = multivitamin; NPC = Nutritional Prevention of Cancer; NSCPS = Nambour Skin Cancer Prevention Study; PHS = Physician's Health Study; REACT = Roche European American Cataract Trial; RECORD = Randomized Evaluation of Calcium or Vitamin D; RR = relative risk; SCPS = Skin Cancer Prevention Study; SELECT = Selenium and Vitamin E Cancer Prevention Trial; SKICAP-AK = Skin Cancer Prevention Trial-Actinic Keratoses; SU.VI.MAX = Supplementation in Vitamins and Mineral Antioxidants Study; WHI = Women's Health Initiative; WHS = Women's Health Study.

Appendix G Figure 1. Relative Risk for Cardiovascular Disease-Related Mortality at Longest Followup Only, by Supplement

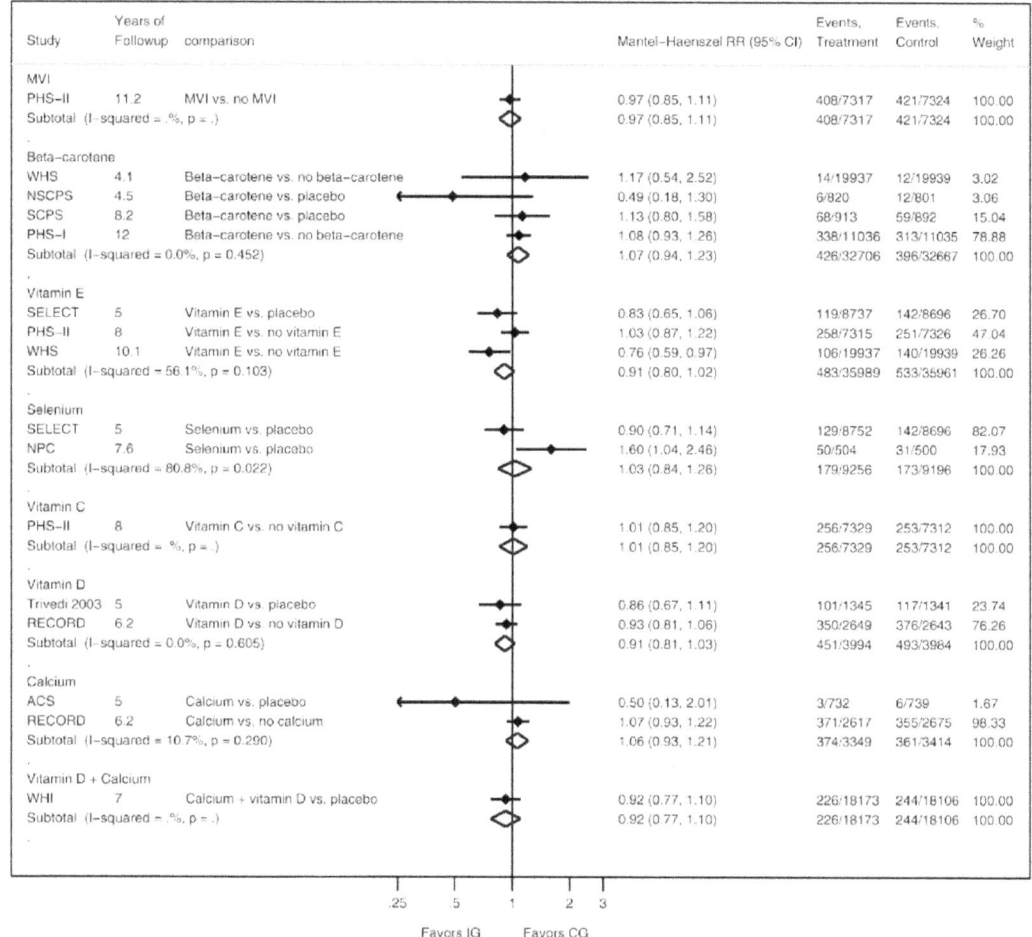

Abbreviations: ACS = Auckland Calcium Study; CG = control group; CI = confidence interval; IG = intervention group; MVI = multivitamin; NPC = Nutritional Prevention of Cancer; NSCPS = Nambour Skin Cancer Prevention Study; PHS = Physician's Health Study; RECORD = Randomized Evaluation of Calcium or Vitamin D; RR = relative risk; SCPS = Skin Cancer Prevention Study; SELECT = Selenium and Vitamin E Cancer Prevention Trial; WHI = Women's Health Initiative; WHS = Women's Health Study.

Appendix G Figure 2. Relative Risk for Myocardial Infarction at Longest Followup Only, by Supplement

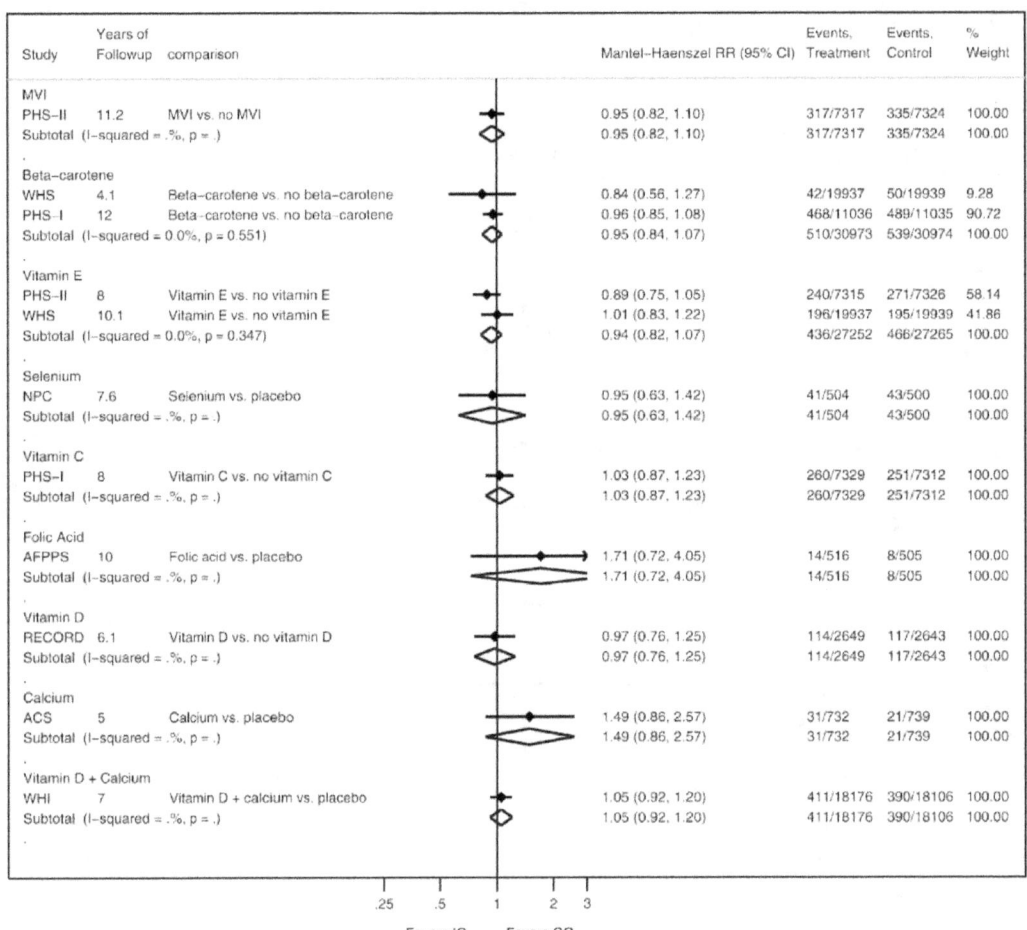

Abbreviations: ACS = Auckland Calcium Study; AFPPS = Aspirin/Folate Polyp Prevention Study; CG = control group; CI = confidence interval; IG = intervention group; MVI = multivitamin; NPC = Nutritional Prevention of Cancer; PHS = Physician's Health Study; RECORD = Randomized Evaluation of Calcium or Vitamin D; RR = relative risk; WHI = Women's Health Initiative; WHS = Women's Health Study.

Appendix G Figure 3. Relative Risk for Stroke at Longest Followup Only, by Supplement

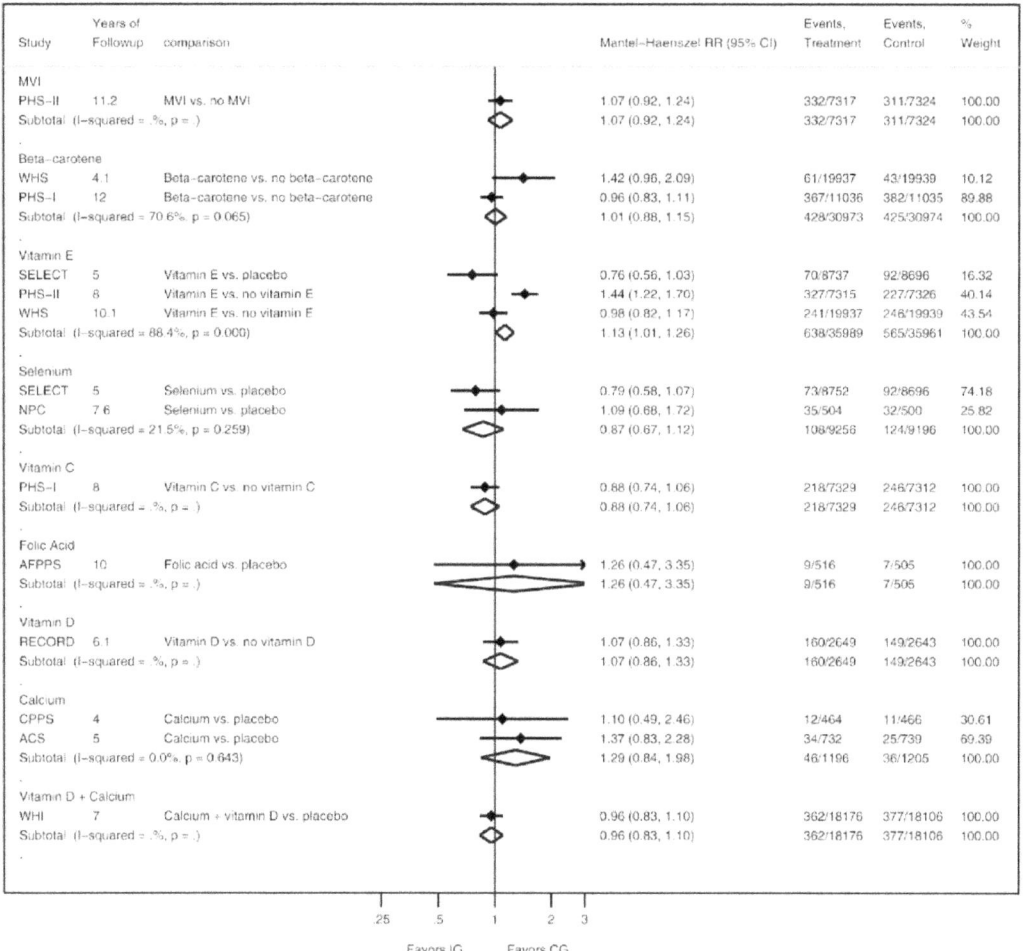

Abbreviations: ACS = Auckland Calcium Study; AFPPS = Aspirin/Folate Polyp Prevention Study; CG = control group; CI = confidence interval; CPPS = Calcium Polyp Prevention Study; IG = intervention group; MVI = multivitamin; NPC = Nutritional Prevention of Cancer; PHS = Physician's Health Study; RECORD = Randomized Evaluation of Calcium or Vitamin D; RR = relative risk; SELECT = Selenium and Vitamin E Cancer Prevention Trial; WHI = Women's Health Initiative; WHS = Women's Health Study.

Appendix G Figure 4. Relative Risk for Any Cancer-Related Mortality at Longest Followup Only, by Supplement

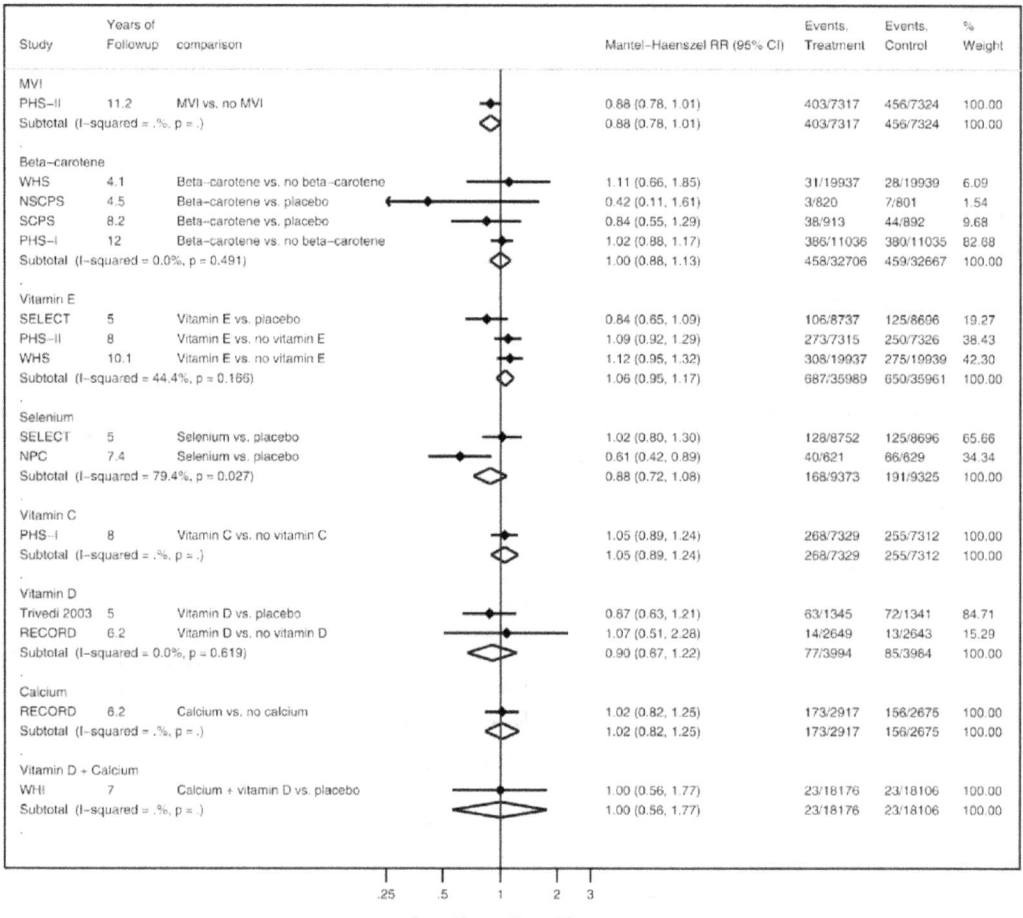

Abbreviations: CG = control group; CI = confidence interval; IG = intervention group; MVI = multivitamin; NPC = Nutritional Prevention of Cancer; NSCPS = Nambour Skin Cancer Prevention Study; PHS = Physician's Health Study; RECORD = Randomized Evaluation of Calcium or Vitamin D; RR = relative risk; SCPS = Skin Cancer Prevention Study; SELECT = Selenium and Vitamin E Cancer Prevention Trial; WHI = Women's Health Initiative; WHS = Women's Health Study.

Appendix G Figure 5. Relative Risk for Lung Cancer at Longest Followup Only, by Supplement

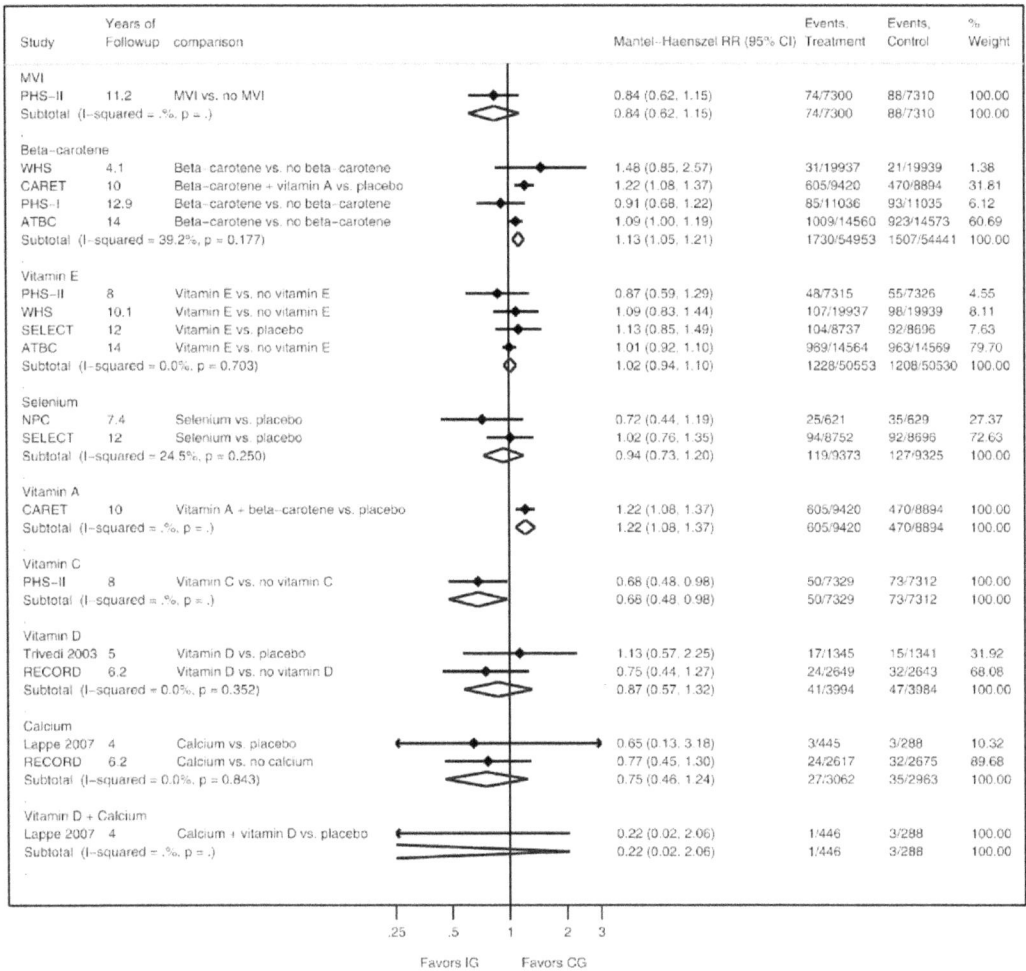

Abbreviations: ATBC = Alpha-Tocopherol Beta-Carotene Cancer Prevention; CARET = Carotene and Retinol Efficacy Trial; CG = control group; CI = confidence interval; IG = intervention group; MVI = multivitamin; NPC = Nutritional Prevention of Cancer; PHS = Physician's Health Study; RECORD = Randomized Evaluation of Calcium or Vitamin D; RR = relative risk; SELECT = Selenium and Vitamin E Cancer Prevention Trial; WHS = Women's Health Study.

Appendix G Figure 6. Odds Ratio for Lung Cancer Mortality at Longest Followup Only, by Supplement

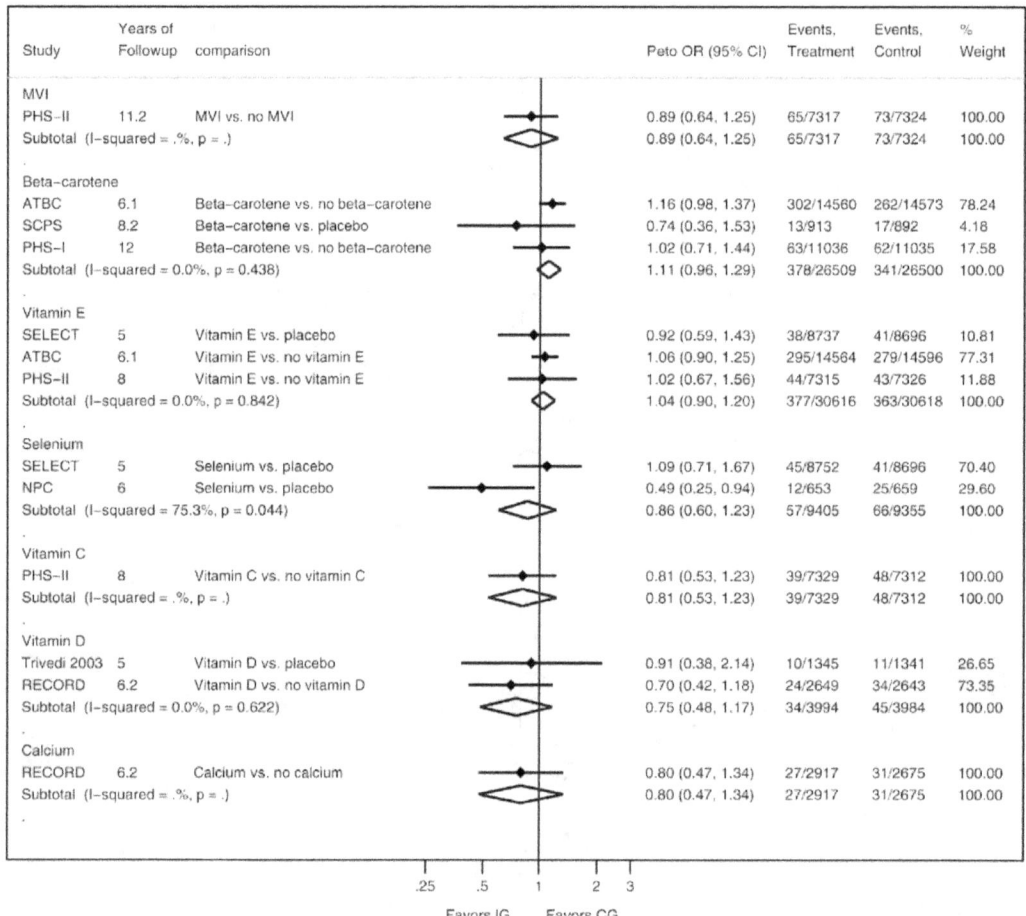

Abbreviations: ATBC = Alpha-Tocopherol Beta-Carotene Cancer Prevention; CG = control group; CI = confidence interval; IG = intervention group; MVI = multivitamin; NPC = Nutritional Prevention of Cancer; OR = odds ratio; PHS = Physician's Health Study; RECORD = Randomized Evaluation of Calcium or Vitamin D; SCPS = Skin Cancer Prevention Study; SELECT = Selenium and Vitamin E Cancer Prevention Trial; WHS = Women's Health Study.

Appendix G Figure 7. Odds Ratio for Colorectal Cancer at Longest Followup Only, by Supplement

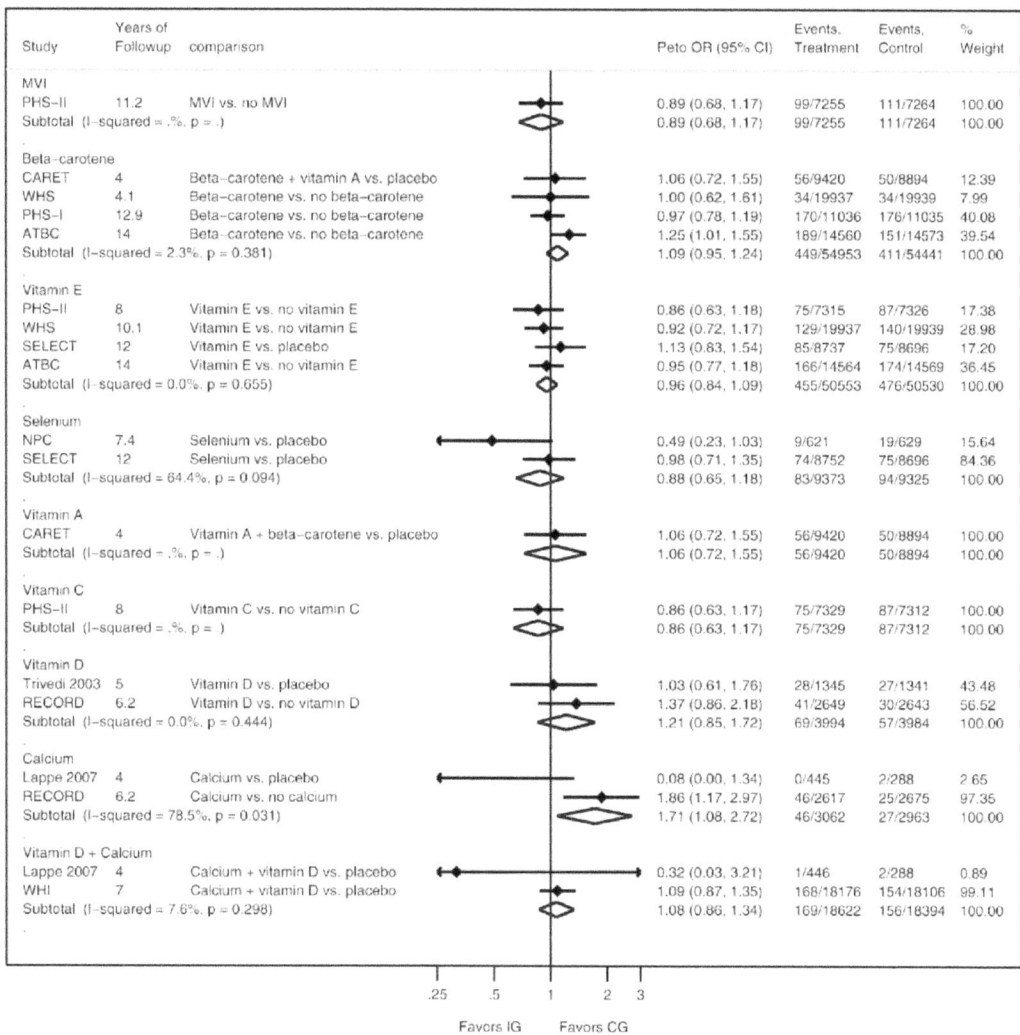

Abbreviations: ATBC = Alpha-Tocopherol Beta-Carotene Cancer Prevention; CARET = Carotene and Retinol Efficacy Trial; CG = control group; CI = confidence interval; IG = intervention group; MVI = multivitamin; NPC = Nutritional Prevention of Cancer; OR = odds ratio; PHS = Physician's Health Study; RECORD = Randomized Evaluation of Calcium or Vitamin D; SELECT = Selenium and Vitamin E Cancer Prevention Trial; WHI = Women's Health Initiative; WHS = Women's Health Study.

Appendix G Figure 8. Odds Ratio for Colorectal Cancer Mortality at Longest Followup Only, by Supplement

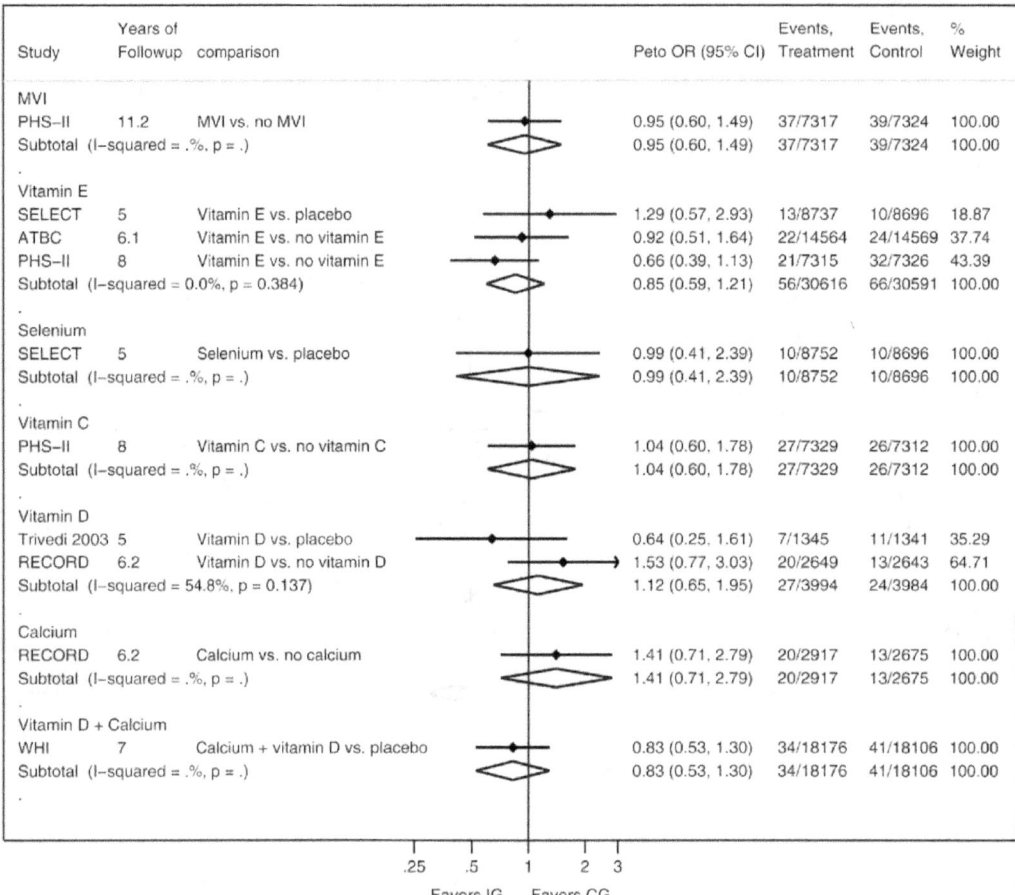

Abbreviations: ATBC = Alpha-Tocopherol Beta-Carotene Cancer Prevention; CG = control group; CI = confidence interval; IG = intervention group; MVI = multivitamin; OR = odds ratio; PHS = Physician's Health Study; RECORD = Randomized Evaluation of Calcium or Vitamin D; SELECT = Selenium and Vitamin E Cancer Prevention Trial; WHI = Women's Health Initiative.

Appendix G Figure 9. Relative Risk for Prostate Cancer at Longest Followup Only, by Supplement

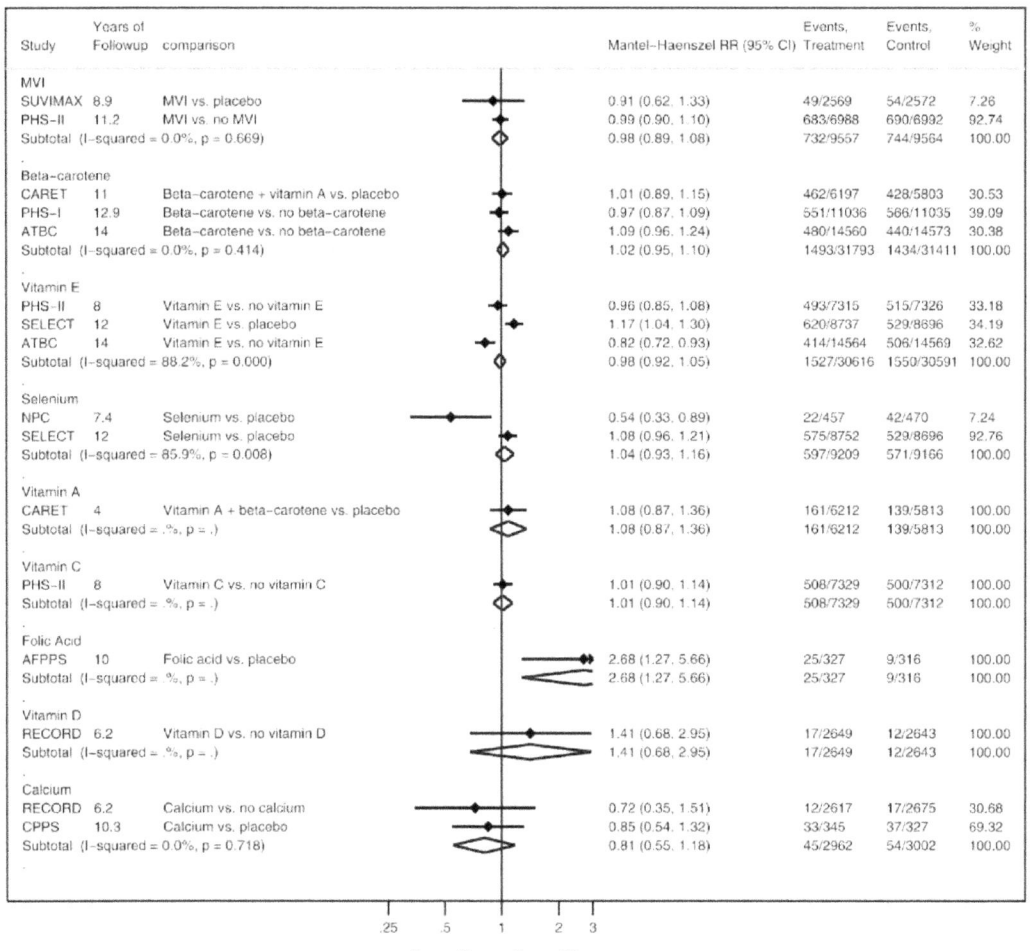

Abbreviations: AFPPS = Aspirin/Folate Polyp Prevention Study; ATBC = Alpha-Tocopherol Beta-Carotene Cancer Prevention; CARET = Carotene and Retinol Efficacy Trial; CG = control group; CI = confidence interval; CPPS = Calcium Polyp Prevention Study; IG = intervention group; MVI = multivitamin; NPC = Nutritional Prevention of Cancer; PHS = Physician's Health Study; RECORD = Randomized Evaluation of Calcium or Vitamin D; RR = relative risk; SELECT = Selenium and Vitamin E Cancer Prevention Trial; SUVIMAX = Supplementation in Vitamins and Mineral Antioxidants Study; WHI = Women's Health Initiative.

Appendix G Figure 10. Odds Ratio for Prostate Cancer Mortality at Longest Followup Only, by Supplement

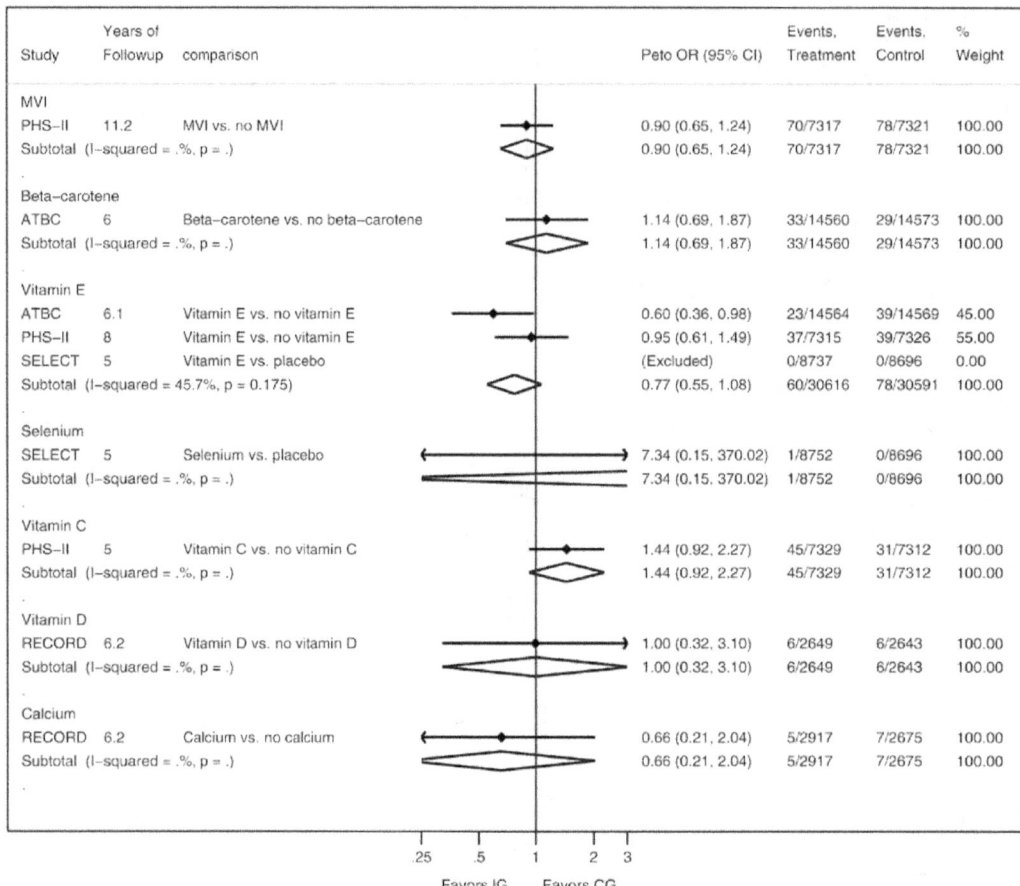

Abbreviations: ATBC = Alpha-Tocopherol Beta-Carotene Cancer Prevention; CG = control group; CI = confidence interval; IG = intervention group; MVI = multivitamin; OR = odds ratio; PHS = Physician's Health Study; RECORD = Randomized Evaluation of Calcium or Vitamin D; SELECT = Selenium and Vitamin E Cancer Prevention Trial.

Appendix G Figure 11. Relative Risk for Breast Cancer at Longest Followup Only, by Supplement

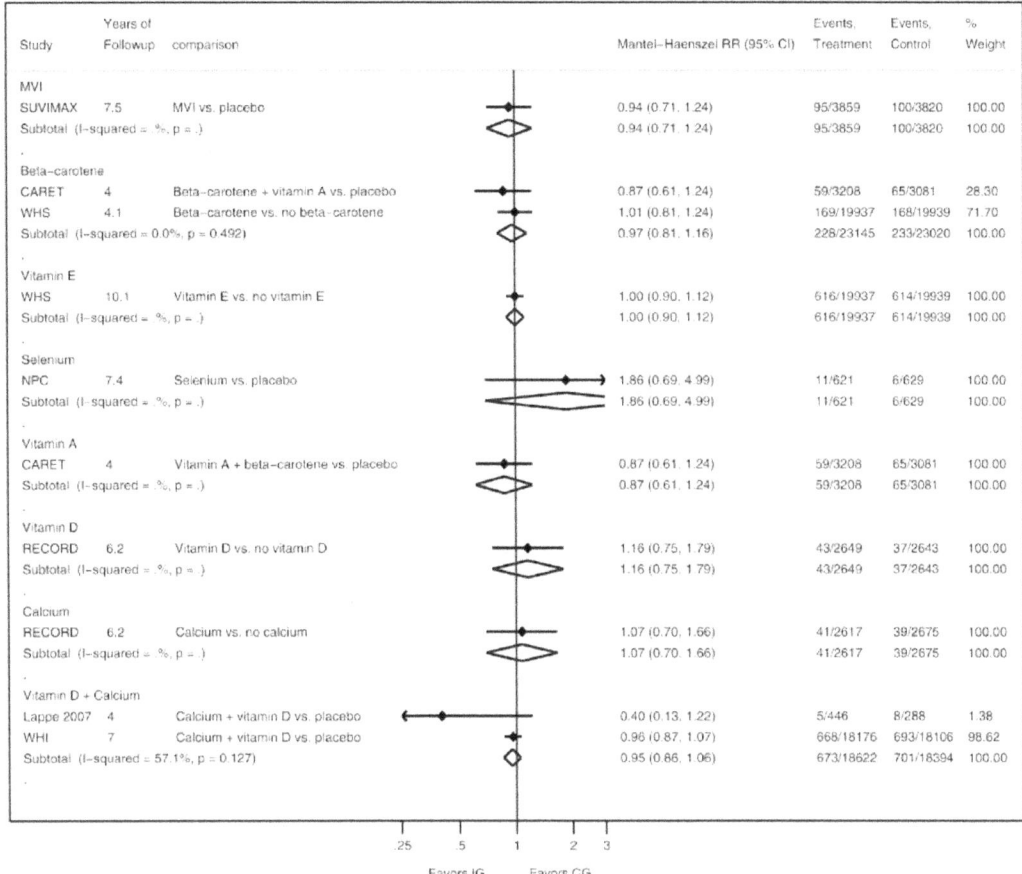

Abbreviations: CARET = Carotene and Retinol Efficacy Trial; CG = control group; CI = confidence interval; IG = intervention group; MVI = multivitamin; PHS = Physician's Health Study; RECORD = Randomized Evaluation of Calcium or Vitamin D; RR = relative risk; SUVIMAX = Supplementation in Vitamins and Mineral Antioxidants Study; WHI = Women's Health Initiative; WHS = Women's Health Study.

Appendix G Figure 12. Odds Ratio for Breast Cancer Mortality at Longest Followup Only, by Supplement

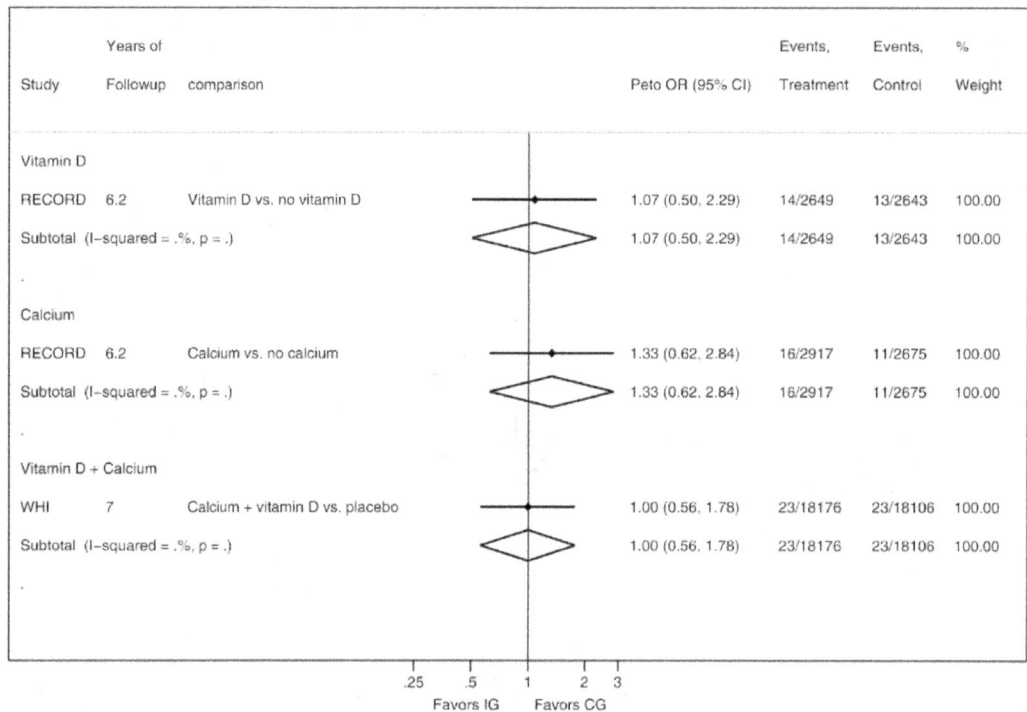

Abbreviations: CG = control group; CI = confidence interval; IG = intervention group; OR = odds ratio; RECORD = Randomized Evaluation of Calcium or Vitamin D; WHI = Women's Health Initiative.

Appendix H Table 1. Unadjusted Relative Risk for All-Cause Mortality at Longest Followup Only, by Supplement

Supplement	Study	DerSimonian and Laird Random Effects Unadjusted RR (95% CI)	Mantel-Haenszel Fixed Effects Unadjusted RR (95% CI)
MVI	REACT	2.98 (0.82, 10.79)	2.98 (0.82, 10.79)
	PHS-II	0.95 (0.89, 1.02)	0.95 (0.89, 1.02)
	SU.VI.MAX	0.88 (0.71, 1.09)	0.88 (0.71, 1.09)
	Subtotal	**0.95 (0.80, 1.11)**	**0.95 (0.89, 1.01)**
Beta-carotene	WHS	1.07 (0.74, 1.55)	1.07 (0.74, 1.55)
	NSCPS	0.51 (0.25, 1.05)	0.51 (0.25, 1.05)
	SCPS	1.03 (0.83, 1.27)	1.03 (0.83, 1.27)
	PHS-I	1.01 (0.93, 1.10)	1.01 (0.93, 1.10)
	ATBC	1.05 (1.02, 1.09)	1.05 (1.02, 1.09)
	Subtotal	**1.04 (0.99, 1.09)**	**1.05 (1.02, 1.08)**
Vitamin E	ASAP	3.00 (0.32, 28.47)	3.00 (0.32, 28.47)
	PHS-II	1.03 (0.94, 1.12)	1.03 (0.94, 1.12)
	WHS	1.03 (0.93, 1.15)	1.03 (0.93, 1.15)
	SELECT	1.01 (0.90, 1.13)	1.01 (0.90, 1.13)
	ATBC	1.01 (0.98, 1.04)	1.01 (0.98, 1.04)
	Subtotal	1.01 (0.98, 1.04)	1.01 (0.98, 1.04)
Selenium	**NPC**	**0.99 (0.78, 1.25)**	**0.98 (0.78, 1.24)**
	SELECT	0.97 (0.87, 1.09)	0.97 (0.87, 1.09)
	Subtotal	0.97 (0.88, 1.08)	0.97 (0.88, 1.08)
Vitamin A	SKICAP-AK	1.15 (0.81, 1.65)	1.15 (0.81, 1.65)
Vitamin C	ASAP	1.00 (0.06, 15.82)	1.00 (0.06, 15.82)
	PHS-II	1.06 (0.97, 1.16)	1.06 (0.97, 1.16)
	Subtotal	1.06 (0.97, 1.16)	1.06 (0.97, 1.16)
Folic Acid	AFPPS	0.52 (0.24, 1.10)	0.52 (0.24, 1.10)
Vitamin D	Trivedi 2003	0.90 (0.77, 1.07)	0.90 (0.77, 1.07)
	RECORD	0.95 (0.88, 1.02)	0.95 (0.88, 1.02)
	Subtotal	**0.94 (0.88, 1.01)**	**0.94 (0.87, 1.01)**
Calcium	CPPS	1.14 (0.65, 1.99)	1.14 (0.65, 1.99)
	ACS	1.18 (0.73, 1.92)	1.18 (0.73, 1.92)
	RECORD	1.03 (0.95, 1.11)	1.03 (0.95, 1.11)
	Subtotal	1.04 (0.96, 1.12)	1.04 (0.96, 1.12)
Vitamin D + Calcium	WHI	0.92 (0.83, 1.01)	0.92 (0.83, 1.01)

Abbreviations: ACS = Auckland Calcium Study; AFPPS = Aspirin/Folate Polyp Prevention Study; ASAP = Antioxidant Supplementation in Atherosclerosis Prevention; ATBC = Alpha-Tocopherol Beta-Carotene Cancer Prevention; CI = confidence interval; CPPS = Calcium Polyp Prevention Study; MVI = multivitamin; NPC = Nutritional Prevention of Cancer; NSCPS = Nambour Skin Cancer Prevention Study; PHS = Physician's Health Study; REACT = Roche European American Cataract Trial; RECORD = Randomized Evaluation of Calcium or Vitamin D; RR = relative risk; SCPS = Skin Cancer Prevention Study; SELECT = Selenium and Vitamin E Cancer Prevention Trial; SKICAP-AK = Skin Cancer Prevention Trial-Actinic Keratoses; SU.VI.MAX = Supplementation in Vitamins and Mineral Antioxidants Study; WHI = Women's Health Initiative; WHS = Women's Health Study.

Appendix H Table 2. Unadjusted Relative Risk for Any Cancer Incidence at Longest Followup Only, by Supplement

Supplement	Study	DerSimonian and Laird Random Effects Unadjusted RR (95% CI)	Mantel-Haenszel Fixed Effects Unadjusted RR (95% CI)
MVI	PHS-II	0.94 (0.87, 1.00)	0.94 (0.87, 1.00)
	SU.VI.MAX	0.97 (0.86, 1.09)	0.97 (0.86, 1.09)
	Subtotal	0.94 (0.89, 1.00)	0.94 (0.89, 1.00)
Beta-carotene	WHS	1.02 (0.89, 1.18)	1.02 (0.89, 1.18)
	PHS-I	0.97 (0.90, 1.04)	0.97 (0.90, 1.04)
	Subtotal	0.98 (0.92, 1.05)	0.98 (0.92, 1.05)
Vitamin E	PHS-II	1.03 (0.95, 1.12)	1.03 (0.95, 1.12)
	WHS	1.01 (0.94, 1.08)	1.01 (0.94, 1.08)
	SELECT	1.07 (0.99, 1.15)	1.07 (0.99, 1.15)
	Subtotal	1.03 (0.99, 1.08)	1.03 (0.99, 1.08)
Selenium	NPC	0.78 (0.62, 0.98)	0.78 (0.62, 0.98)
	SELECT	1.02 (0.94, 1.10)	1.02 (0.94, 1.10)
	Subtotal	**0.91 (0.70, 1.18)**	**0.99 (0.92, 1.06)**
Vitamin C	PHS-II	1.00 (0.92, 1.09)	1.00 (0.92, 1.09)
Folic Acid	AFPPS	1.65 (1.09, 2.51)	1.65 (1.09, 2.51)
Vitamin D	Trivedi 2003	1.08 (0.89, 1.31)	1.08 (0.89, 1.31)
	RECORD	1.04 (0.91, 1.19)	1.04 (0.91, 1.19)
	Subtotal	1.05 (0.94, 1.18)	1.05 (0.94, 1.18)
Calcium	CPPS	0.72 (0.97, 1.37)	0.72 (0.97, 1.37)
	Lappe 2007	0.55 (0.29, 1.03)	0.55 (0.29, 1.03)
	RECORD	1.08 (0.94, 1.23)	1.08 (0.94, 1.23)
	Subtotal	1.03 (0.90, 1.17)	1.03 (0.90, 1.17)
Vitamin D + Calcium	WHI	0.98 (0.92, 1.05)	0.98 (0.92, 1.05)
	Lappe 2007	0.42 (0.21, 0.83)	0.42 (0.21, 0.83)
	Subtotal	**0.69 (0.30, 1.57)**	**0.98 (0.91, 1.04)**

Abbreviations: AFPPS = Aspirin/Folate Polyp Prevention Study; CI = confidence interval; CPPS = Calcium Polyp Prevention Study; MVI = multivitamin; NPC = Nutritional Prevention of Cancer; PHS = Physician's Health Study; RECORD = Randomized Evaluation of Calcium or Vitamin D; RR = relative risk; SELECT = Selenium and Vitamin E Cancer Prevention Trial; SU.VI.MAX = Supplementation in Vitamins and Mineral Antioxidants Study; WHI = Women's Health Initiative; WHS = Women's Health Study.